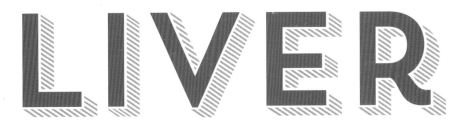

HEALTHY
LIVER

Dr CRIS BEER

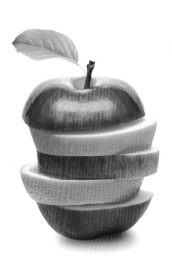

ROCKPOOL
PUBLISHING

About Dr Cris Beer

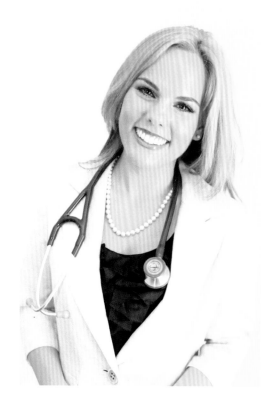

*BBioMedSci, MBBS (hons), FRACGP,
member ACNEM, member AIMA,
Cert IV in Fitness*

As an expert in nutritional medicine Dr Cris specialises not just in the prevention and treatment of illnesses, but in the attaining of optimum health. By employing simple lifestyle and holistic medicine strategies, Dr Cris believes that restoration of health and vitality can be achieved by anyone. Dr Cris holds qualifications in medicine, biomedical science, integrative and nutritional medicine, health coaching, as well as personal fitness training. She was the health consultant for *The Biggest Loser Retreat* and is sought by the media for regular commentary on radio, TV, newspaper columns, as well as print magazines. She currently practises at *The Medical Sanctuary* on the Gold Coast as a registered medical doctor helping patients every day. For more information go to **drcris.com.au**

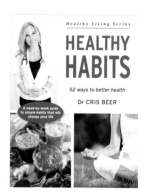

More books by Dr Cris...
ISBN: 978-1-925017-54-0

Healthy Habits – 52 Ways to Better Health is an easy-to-read book offering an effective 'habit-a-week' approach to good health, energy, and optimum body weight.

Available at all good bookstores or online at www.rockpoolpublishing.com.au

Contents

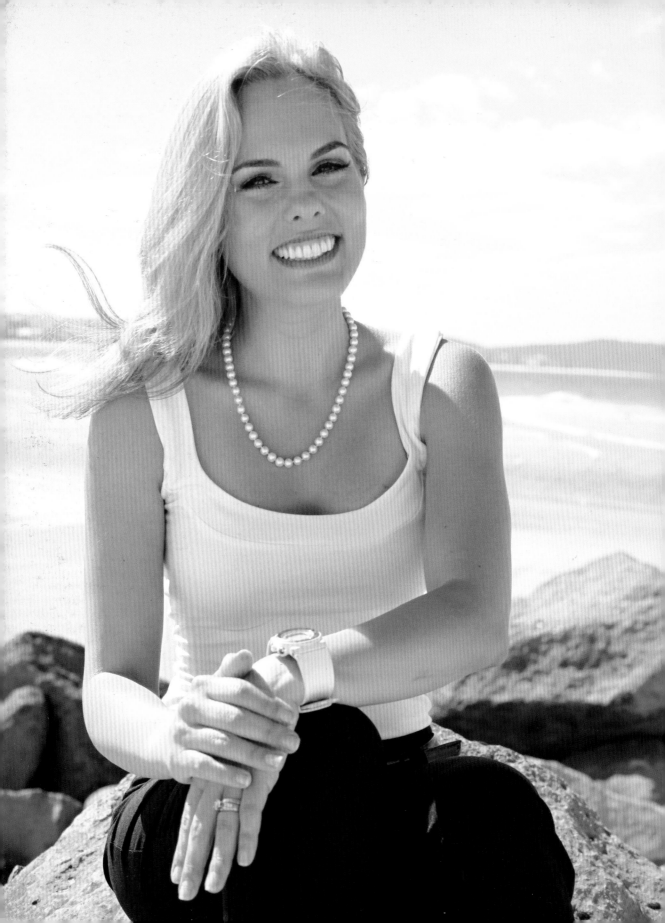

►►►

WHO NEEDS A HEALTHY LIVER?

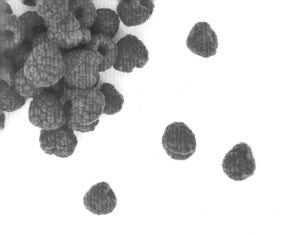

For the first few years that I worked as a general practitioner I had underestimated the liver's significant role in the general wellbeing of my patients. I had learnt that the liver was important from a physiological point of view and that it helped to keep us alive, but I hadn't fully considered how it keeps us feeling well on a day-to-day basis.

I had been taught how to detect liver-function abnormalities in blood testing and how to feel for an enlarged or tender liver – all signs of obvious and severe liver damage. But as for understanding liver damaged well before any obvious clinical signs begin to show, I was completely in the dark. I had seen severe liver damage from chronic alcoholism and from liver disease such as hepatitis, but the subtler symptoms and signs of liver impairment was something I was not adept at detecting. It wasn't until I started

practising holistic medicine that I realised the big part the liver plays in a patient's ability to get well and stay well.

Many patients who present to my clinic are struggling to lose weight despite exercising regularly and eating relatively healthily. They often have fluid retention, hormone issues such as low libido, and generally feel tired and unwell. The answer for these patients is not to eat less and move more, as popular advice would suggest, but rather to investigate the deeper physiological issues in that patient's body. This physiological disturbance is often rooted in poor liver health, as a cause or consequence of the patient's lifestyle choices, genetics, infection and/or something known as environmental overload. These will be explained further in the section on 'Liver Haters' but for now let's look at who can benefit from having a healthy liver.

Who Benefits from a Healthy Liver?

This is really a rhetorical question because everyone can benefit from having a healthy liver! If you value your wellbeing and want to feel healthy and energetic then looking after your liver is key. In particular, the following issues may indicate compromised liver health:

- ✓ Struggling to lose weight

- ✓ Carrying weight around your mid-section

- ✓ Feeling tired despite getting a good night's sleep (including those with chronic fatigue syndrome and/or fibromyalgia)

- ✓ Feeling bloated

- ✓ Unexplained itchy skin, especially at night

- ✓ Dark circles under your eyes

- ✓ Excess fluid, especially around your ankles

- ✓ A coating on your tongue

- ✓ Bruising easily

- ✓ Having a poor immune system

- ✓ Have blotchy skin

- ✓ Frequent headaches

- ✓ Gallbladder issues such as gallstones

- ✓ High cholesterol levels or high blood pressure

- ✓ Having been diagnosed with fatty liver

- ✓ Having been diagnosed with metabolic syndrome

- ✓ Liver function abnormalities detected in blood testing

- ✓ Consistently drinking too much alcohol or binge drinking

- ✓ Having taken regular pain-killer medications, anti-depressants or other mood stabilising medications, the oral contraceptive pill, hormone-replacement therapy, epilepsy medications, antibiotics, or cholesterol-lowering medications over a period of time

- ✓ Having hepatitis or cirrhosis (infection-related or alcohol-related)

As you can see, many of us would fit into the category of needing a healthier liver based on some of the more common symptoms presented above. You may not even realise your liver is your key health issue as liver health can deteriorate gradually and almost unnoticeably at first. It is not until symptoms begin interfering with a person's quality of life that they seek help. Hopefully at this point liver deterioration can be addressed and health can return.

This was definitely my case in my mid-twenties when I found myself struggling with feeling constantly bloated and tired. Even though I was considered to have a normal body weight for my frame, I was struggling to lose a few extra kilograms around my mid-section. This was very frustrating as I was exercising five days a week and doing what I thought were 'all the right things'. I felt overwhelmed most of the time, irritated, and retained fluid, which I noticed particularly at the end of the day when my rings no longer seemed to fit on my fingers. I scratched my arms, palms and legs most nights with an unexplained itch that seemed to resolve in the daytime. I couldn't see any signs of eczema or dermatitis and moisturised regularly, just in case this itch was due to dry skin, but that did not seem to make any difference.

Despite having a relatively healthy diet and being a non-smoker and non-drinker, I had elevated cholesterol levels. I was referred by my local doctor to a heart specialist, who shrugged his shoulders and suggested that my cholesterol level was probably a result of genetics, rather than my lifestyle.

What I discovered, though, several years later, was that my liver was the issue. A combination of some poor lifestyle choices, a higher-dose oral contraceptive pill (that I had been on since I was 14, for acne), and some genetic susceptibilities, had overloaded my liver and elevated my bad cholesterol levels. Once these factors were addressed my cholesterol levels and my health returned to normal. I no longer felt tired or struggled to lose weight around my middle; I no longer felt irritated or scratched my skin at night (to my husband's relief!). I just wished I had realised that my liver health was my main issue beforehand – it would have saved me years of feeling terrible!

I'm sure my story is not unique – perhaps you are feeling exactly the same way. Tired, struggling with your weight and just simply not feeling great. The answer lies in addressing your liver health.

How Will This Book Help You?

What I learnt in my journey to improving my liver health, and ultimately my overall health and wellbeing, was that there are some key steps to follow in order to restore the liver to its original function. These steps are based on holistic health principles, with the best of both conventional and complementary wisdoms brought together. This book offers these steps in an easy-to-follow format so that each step is manageable

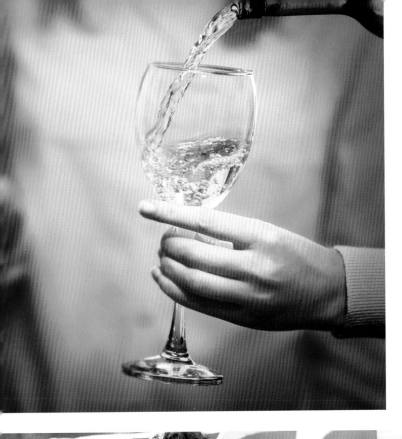
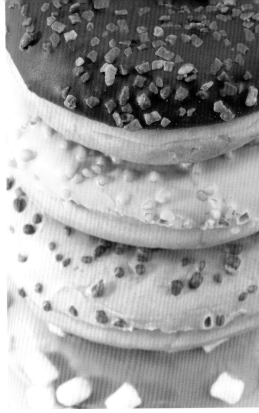
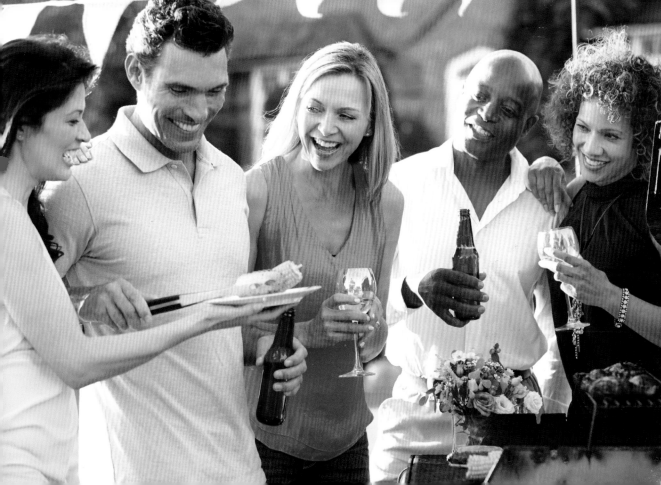

and able to be implemented into busy lives. It is easy to feel overwhelmed in today's society with such an abundance of health information available at our fingertips and often we become paralysed, unable to act – not knowing which way to go. In this book I hope to help you on the path to gaining a healthy liver. The key to making change is one step at a time.

The first step is to understand where your health lies. This is sometimes difficult to quantify as the experience of health is relative for each person based on their previous experiences and expectations. This is also true of liver health, which is perhaps even more difficult to pinpoint given the liver is an organ often not immediately associated with the symptoms listed. To help you gauge where your liver health may stand, I have put together a questionnaire in the section, 'Know Your Liver'. From this questionnaire you will get a Liver Health Score. The higher the score the more likely your health issues stem from poor-liver health.

The section titled 'Your Liver Detox Plan' will then outline a specific plan to restore your liver to healthy working order. Your Liver Health Score will help determine which particular supportive strategies

you may need to incorporate into Your Liver Detox as well as the recommended duration of the Detox. Each step of this Detox is laid out clearly so that you never need to feel overwhelmed or confused.

Once you have completed Your Liver Detox the goal is to maintain liver health. If you happen to splurge one weekend with way too much indulging, then follow the steps outlined in 'Your Post-Party Detox'. This will help you get back on track fast. Both Your Liver Detox and Your Post-Party Detox are summarised in the 'Easy Reference Guide' section of this book to print/take a photo of for future reference and as a reminder of what I have covered.

The final section of this book is a description of seven interesting liver cases that I have seen in clinical practice. The purpose of this section is to help consolidate what you have learnt and to know that you are not alone! By reading others' experiences we can learn something about our own liver health and feel comfortable to take positive steps forward.

So use *Healthy Liver* as your guide to walk you through those steps and discover what it feels like to have optimal liver health. The proof is in the results you experience. If you follow the advice in this book you will regain your health and vitality. You will feel years younger and have more energy than you have had in years.

Will the Detox Be Hard or Time Consuming to Follow?

The strategies suggested have been developed with the busy person in mind. They are easy to follow and not time consuming to implement. Each step is based on practical, sensible and proven strategies not intended to be burdensome or have severe restrictions or rules to follow. It is easier to make changes to your health and lifestyle if you have the support of family members or an accountability person, who can help you to stay focussed. Encouraging others to come along the journey with you to discover great liver health will also help you to stay motivated and allow you to share these health benefits with others.

Will It Take Long to Restore an Unhealthy Liver?

The time it takes to restore optimal liver function will depend on how damaged your liver is and for how long your liver health has been neglected. Be reassured,

though, the liver is a remarkably hardy organ that is able to regenerate even in cases of significant damage. Your Liver Health Score will gauge how damaged your liver is, which will determine how long you need to do the Detox for.

Your Liver Detox incorporates a 7-Day Liver Detox Diet. This is designed to be achievable for most and allows individuals to relax a little with their Detox on the weekends. It can be repeated week after week, if desired, or as required, based on your Liver Health Score, to achieve optimal liver health. For minimal liver damage, seven days may be enough to restore liver health. This diet may be repeated several times throughout the year as a 'reset', for example, following Christmas – a time of indulgence with food and drink. There is no harm in following Your Liver Detox long-term as it is based on a balanced diet.

Can Anyone Do the Liver Detox?

The answer to this is yes. Your Liver Detox is a healthy, balanced approach to detoxing the liver and restoring liver health. It is not extreme or based on fad diets. You will still be able to work and function normally on this plan. In fact, you will find that you will be able to carry out your usual activities with more vigour and energy than previously.

I would recommend consulting your doctor first before undertaking Your Liver Detox if you suffer from diabetes or any other major chronic health condition such as hepatitis. This is to gauge response and to make sure medication dosages still apply. Keep in mind that Your Liver Detox does not replace medical treatment in the form of medications or other treatments as recommended by your local doctor. Saying that, many of my patients have found that the dosages of certain medications, such as cholesterol and diabetes medications, can be lowered once their liver health is restored. Always consult your doctor, first, however, before weaning off or changing any medications.

Pregnant and breast-feeding women can undertake the Detox with the exclusion of the recommended supportive supplements. The safety of these supplements during pregnancy and breast-feeding are unknown. It is also recommended that if you are pregnant or breast-feeding to consult your doctor or nutritionist first before undertaking the Detox as these are times when further nutritional intake is required. Your doctor or nutritionist can ensure that no deficiencies arise.

Children over the age of 12 may also undertake the Detox if their liver health is of concern. This is best done in consultation with your child's paediatrician or local doctor.

So, your journey to great liver health now begins. To start that journey let us first take a closer look at what the liver actually does so that we can understand what might be happening to our liver when we start to feel unwell.

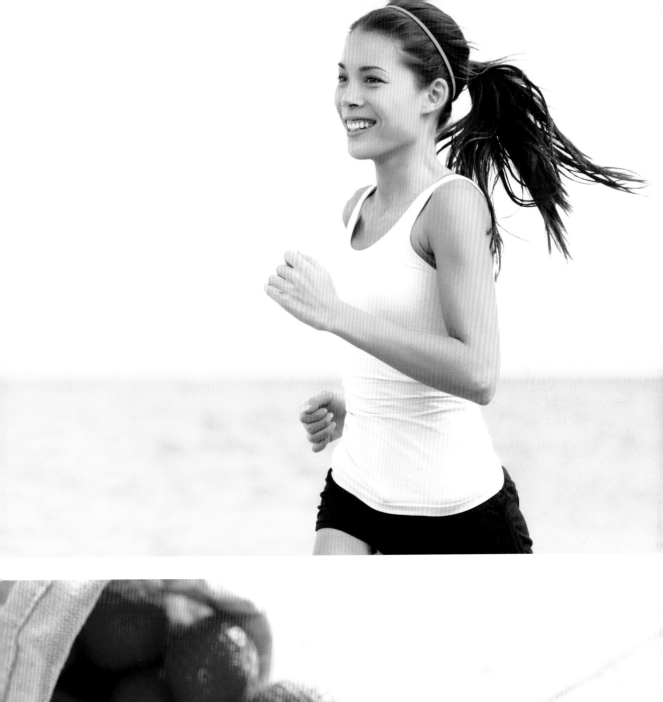
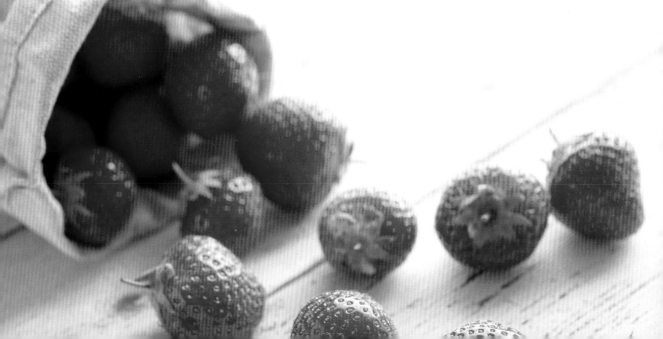

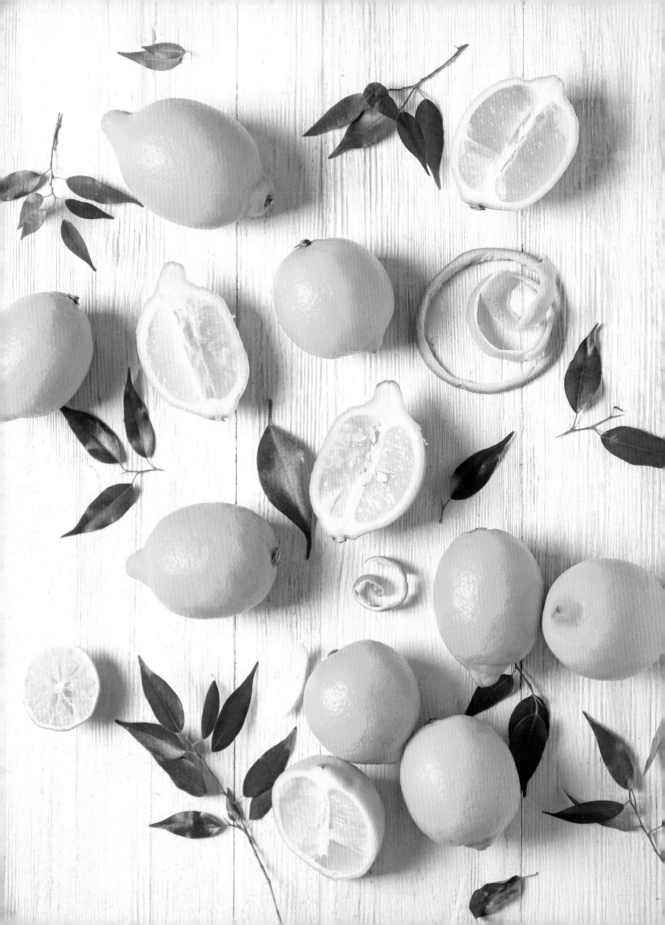

▶ ▶ ▷

INTRO
TO LIVER
HEALTH

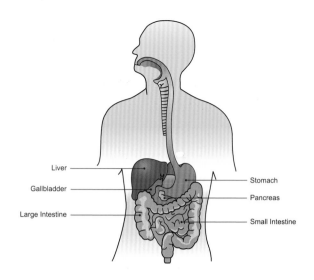

Liver
Gallbladder
Large Intestine

Stomach
Pancreas
Small Intestine

- ✓ Have a normal metabolism and healthy body weight for your frame

- ✓ Have normal, healthy cholesterol levels in your blood

- ✓ Not have any coating on your tongue

- ✓ Have a healthy immune system

- ✓ Not bruise easily

Your liver is essential. It has over 500 imperative functions to help keep your body healthy. However, its role in our general wellbeing can easily be overlooked. In order to get well and stay well, liver health needs to be addressed. In today's society our liver can really take a hit through our lifestyles and via general environment insults (as we will discuss further in the chapter on 'Liver Haters').

A healthy liver will complement other body systems that are functioning optimally, as the body works as a whole. How other organs impact on liver health and vice versa is touched on below and further discussed in the 'Your Liver Detox Plan' section. If your liver is healthy you will:

- ✓ Feel energetic

- ✓ Have clear eyes with no dark circles under your eyes

- ✓ Have clear skin

Where Is My Liver?

Most people have a vague idea where their liver is located. It is found on the upper right side of the abdomen, just below the diaphragm and underneath the ribs on that side. It is the largest internal organ and weighs around 1.5kg. It is boarded by the intestines, pancreas and stomach.

The liver receives a blood supply from the general circulation as well as directly from our digestive tract. Blood supply from our digestive tract carries food particles, medicines that we have ingested and micro-organisms (bugs found in our food and water supplies) that have been absorbed in the intestines to the liver. These substances are then sorted by at least one of the liver's amazing internal processes.

What Exactly Does My Liver Do?

Your liver is essentially your internal chemical – and nutrient – processing factory. It enables chemical reactions that rid the body of toxins and internal cellular waste products, and it processes food nutrients to help maintain a constant supply of these nutrients to our body's various organs and tissues.

Let's look a little further at some of the main functions of the liver so that we can understand what is happening to this organ when we start to feel unwell. The liver:

- Rids the body of toxins such as medications, alcohol and other

potentially harmful substances in our diet and environment. The liver does this in two stages (known as phase 1 and phase 2). These phases require the assistance of certain nutrients, vitamins and minerals found in our diet, which we will discuss further in the chapter titled 'Liver Lovers'.

The purpose of detoxification is to convert toxins into harmless substances able to be eliminated from the body (in faeces, urine or sweat) via various other organs as shown in the diagram below.

As we can see from this diagram there are four other organ systems that work together with the liver to detoxify the

LIVER DETOXIFICATION PROCESS

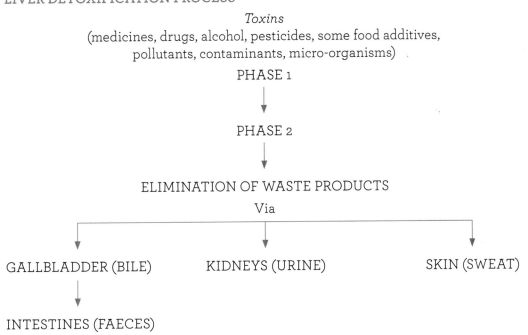

Toxins
(medicines, drugs, alcohol, pesticides, some food additives, pollutants, contaminants, micro-organisms)

PHASE 1

↓

PHASE 2

↓

ELIMINATION OF WASTE PRODUCTS
Via

GALLBLADDER (BILE)   KIDNEYS (URINE)   SKIN (SWEAT)

↓

INTESTINES (FAECES)

body – the gallbladder, our intestines, kidneys and our skin. These organs also need to be functioning optimally in order for the liver to do its job effectively. Ways to assist the function of these organs will be outlined further in the section 'Your Liver Detox Plan'.

Along with detoxification the liver also undertakes the following functions:

- Produces bile (stored in the gallbladder, which is attached to the liver and emptied into the intestines) that is used to help break down dietary fats and absorb the fat-soluble vitamins A, D, E and K in our diet. The liver is able to store these vitamins for gradual use by the body as well as vitamin B12 and the minerals iron and copper.

- Filters the blood and removes degraded blood cells as well as invading bacteria

- Breaks down any unwanted or harmful hormones

- Converts carbohydrates in the diet into glucose for instant energy and stores the excess glucose into glycogen (the stored form of glucose) so if blood sugar levels drop glycogen is converted back into glucose to restore blood sugar balance

- Synthesises cholesterols and the production of lipoproteins, which transport cholesterol including low-density lipoprotein (LDL) and high-density lipoprotein (HDL) throughout the body. Cholesterol is an essential component of our cell walls and is also used in hormone production.

- Metabolises fat and helps to regulate body-fat stores. When energy levels are low, between meals and during exercise, the liver can convert fatty acids into an alternative energy supply known as ketones.

- Produces body proteins, including hormones, from amino-acid building blocks. The liver is also able to convert the excess protein in amino acids into fat for storage. If extra energy is needed by your body, the liver will convert amino acids into glucose.

- Regulates blood clotting to assist healing and prevent internal bleeding

- Produces immune system cells used in fighting infections

With these functions of the liver clearly outlined it is easy to see how important it is for our health and how important it is to look after it. So how well *is* your liver functioning? In the next chapter we will discuss common symptoms of poor liver health and see what your Liver Health Score actually is.

Liver Functions

Removes potentially toxic byproducts of certain medications.

Prevents shortages of nutrients by storing vitamins, minerals and sugar.

Metabolises, or breaks down, nutrients from food to produce energy, when needed.

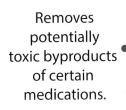

Produces most proteins needed by the body.

Helps your body fight infection by removing bacteria from the blood and also produces immune cells used to fight infection.

Produces most of the substances that regulate blood clotting.

Produces bile, a compound needed to digest fat and to absorb vitamins A, D, E and K.

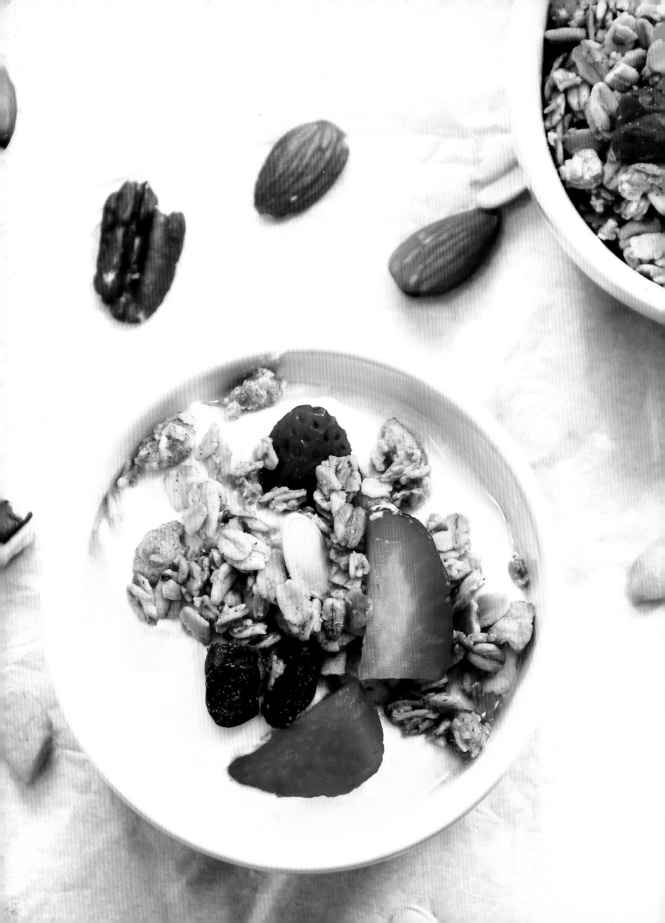

KNOW YOUR LIVER

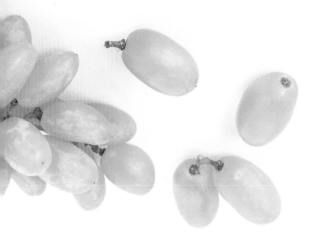

From the previous chapter explaining the vital functions of the liver it is easy to see why you start to accumulate harmful toxins in your body when your liver is damaged. You cannot process food nutrients as efficiently and, as a result, your metabolism and immune system are compromised.

These effects result in a range of symptoms depending on the severity of the liver damage such as:

- ✓ Fatigue

- ✓ General malaise (feeling unwell)

- ✓ Nausea

- ✓ Vomiting

- ✓ Unexplained itching, which is worse at night

- ✓ Diarrhoea

- ✓ Appetite loss

- ✓ Bloated abdomen

- ✓ Swollen ankles

- ✓ Abdominal pain under right side of ribcage

- ✓ Easy bruising

- ✓ Reduced immunity resulting in potentially more infections such as head colds

- ✓ Reddened skin, especially palms

- ✓ Jaundice (the skin or whites of the eyes turn yellow)

- ✓ Dark urine

- ✓ Fever

- ✓ Anaemia

Let's now determine how healthy your liver is by taking the following Liver Health Questionnaire. This will give you a score, your Liver Health Score, from zero to the highest possible score of fifty-four. Remember the higher your score the more likely you will need to address your liver health. Don't be fearful of what your Liver Health Score result might be, as some simple changes to lifestyle and diet will help you get back on track – in particular, Your Liver Detox.

Your Liver Health Score

Complete the following Liver Health Questionnaire to find out your Liver Health Score. This score will then be used to gauge your current liver health and will direct you to the optimal Detox plan in order to begin the healing process. Score the following questions from zero, where a symptom does not apply to you, to three, where you experience that particular symptom daily.

Liver Health Questionnaire

	Nil	Sometimes	Often	Daily
You feel tired despite getting a good night's sleep	0	1	2	3
Your skin becomes itchy at night	0	1	2	3
You have dark circles under your eyes	0	1	2	3
You experience pain in your right upper abdomen	0	1	2	3
You have dark-coloured urine	0	1	2	3
You have pale chalky stools	0	1	2	3
You bruise easily	0	1	2	3
You have noticed red freckle-like skin spots appear	0	1	2	3
You find it hard to lose weight	0	1	2	3
You have reddened skin, particularly on your palms	0	1	2	3
You have a yellow tinge to your skin or to the whites of your eyes	0	1	2	3
You often feel nauseated	0	1	2	3
You have swollen feet and/or legs	0	1	2	3
You often have diarrhoea	0	1	2	3
You have lost your appetite	0	1	2	3
You have a coating on your tongue	0	1	2	3
You drink three or more alcoholic drinks in one sitting	0	1	2	3
You experience frequent headaches	0	1	2	3

Now add up your Liver Health Score and see which of the below three categories applies to you. Keep in mind that the higher your score the more you need to address your liver health. However, if your Liver Health Score is very high it may not mean you are extremely ill or have a definite disease of the liver, but that this is an opportunity to address your diet and lifestyle before a serious illness does present.

Less than 5 – Unlikely Liver Damage

If you scored less than five then you are very unlikely to have any liver damage. You will still benefit from following the Detox, however, as this is a plan that will help to improve and maintain anyone's overall health. Perhaps consider following Your Liver Detox Plan after times of indulgence such as Easter and Christmas, or just to reset your health at the start or middle of the year.

Between 6 and 18 – Mild Liver Damage Possible

If you scored between six and eighteen, then you could have mild liver damage. This may have been caused by a number of factors such as regular alcohol consumption, toxin exposure, infection or medication use. These factors are explained further in the next section on

'Liver Haters'. Following Your Liver Detox will definitely benefit your health and it is worth undertaking the 7-Day Liver Detox Diet component of Your Liver Detox for the recommended minimum period of one full week.

You may choose to complete another seven days of the 7-Day Liver Detox Diet following this, either consecutively or with a weekend off in between. You can repeat this process for as long as you like or until your symptoms have eased and your liver health has improved.

Between 19 and 39 – Moderate Liver Damage Likely

If you scored between nineteen and thirty-nine then you are likely to have a moderate level of liver damage. This may have been caused by long-term excessive alcohol intake that has led to alcoholic hepatitis, strong medication use (such as higher dose painkillers), as a result of fatty liver disease or metabolic syndrome or as a result of viral hepatitis (such as hepatitis C or B infection).

It is recommended that you undertake several rounds of the 7-Day Liver Detox Diet until your symptoms abate. With this level of liver damage, it is likely that abnormalities will appear in liver function blood tests and/or scans with an ultrasound machine. In this case you are likely to need to continue to undertake the Detox until these test results return to normal. Your local doctor will be the best person to guide you on your progress as you continue with Your Liver Detox.

You may break on the weekends from Your Liver Detox, but for best results, based on the current level of your liver damage, it would be recommended to only break for a day at most. Based on clinical experience, the amount of time required to significantly improve your liver function is four to six weeks, the exception being viral hepatitis, whereby the Detox does not replace medical treatment but does supplement it. The improvement in viral hepatitis will depend on several factors such as ongoing damage from the virus, lifestyle factors, and effectiveness of medication. Your Liver Detox Plan modifies the lifestyle factor component and thereby may aid recovery from viral hepatitis.

A score of 40 or more – Severe Liver Damage Likely

If you scored forty or more then you are likely to have a severe level of liver damage. This may have been caused by chronic excessive alcohol consumption that has led to severe alcoholic hepatitis

or even cirrhosis of the liver (explained further in the section on 'Liver Haters'), from severe forms of fatty liver disease or metabolic syndrome, or as a result of viral hepatitis (such as hepatitis C or B infection), or from long-term use of medications known to damage the liver such as certain anti-depressants.

It is recommended that you continue Your Liver Detox for at least eight to ten weeks. It is also recommended that with this level of liver damage that you do not break on the weekends from the 7-Day Liver Detox Diet but undertake it continuously until your liver functioning has returned to normal.

A Word About Your Liver Health Score

It is important to note that the symptoms listed in the questionnaire are non-specific when isolated from liver damage and it is the cumulative score of having multiple symptoms that are suggestive of liver damage. It is difficult to say for certain how much liver damage you may have sustained but your Liver Health Score gives us a clue as to your liver health and helps to guide your healing process. A full medical diagnosis of your liver health is recommended to supplement your Liver Health Score.

Keep in mind that some individuals who have significant underlying liver damage may in fact experience very few symptoms or even none at all[1]. This could be due to individual differences in the way we perceive and experience health and the amazing regenerative ability of the liver, which can be a very forgiving organ, of course to a certain degree.

If you answer yes to any of the following, even though you may not be experiencing any symptoms, your liver health is likely to be compromised. I suggest in this case that you follow Your Liver Detox Plan as your health will greatly benefit from it.

	YES/NO
Have gallbladder issues such as gallstones	
Have high cholesterol levels or blood pressure	
Have been diagnosed with fatty liver disease	
Have been diagnosed with metabolic syndrome	
Have had liver function abnormalities detected in blood testing	
Have taken regular painkiller medications, anti-depressants or other mood-stabilising medications, the oral contraceptive pill, hormone-replacement therapy, epilepsy medications, antibiotics, or cholesterol-lowering medications	
Have been diagnosed with hepatitis or cirrhosis (infection-related or alcohol related)	

As you can see from the list above it is important to go ahead and have a full liver health check-up with your doctor. This will detect any underlying liver health issues, which may appear normal from a symptom point of view but can be very abnormal from a pathology point of view.

Your Liver Check-Up

Having a full liver check-up by your local doctor completes the picture of your liver health and will confirm your Liver Health Score.

Provided is an outline of common tools your local doctor will utilise to determine the health of your liver. Many of these are routine, relatively non-invasive and worth undertaking. Once you have had some tests, compare your results with the interpretation of common liver testing as outlined below.

The following tests may be completed during a liver check-up:

- **Physical examination** – your doctor will feel your abdomen gently to detect whether your liver is enlarged or tender (signs of liver damage). They will also ask you to take deep breaths to detect whether this elicits tenderness in your right upper abdomen (a sign of gallbladder disease such as gallstones).

- Blood tests – your doctor will undertake a basic liver function blood test. This detects the levels of liver enzymes and jaundice ('yellowness'), which will help your doctor assess the protein producing capability of the liver. Along

with an elevation in liver enzymes, a rise in ferritin (iron stores), cholesterol and blood sugar levels indicates liver damage. Sometimes blood tests do not reflect the fact that liver damage is in its early stages, however.

You can interpret your liver function testing by looking at the following tables. The first table outlines normal laboratory reference values for standard liver testing. The second table outlines common liver problems and abnormalities that may be seen on laboratory liver testing.

Typical Laboratory Liver Test

Liver Tests	Reference Range of Normal Results
Albumin	34–48
Total Bilirubin	2–24
GGT	<60
ALP	30–110
ALT	< 55
AST	< 45

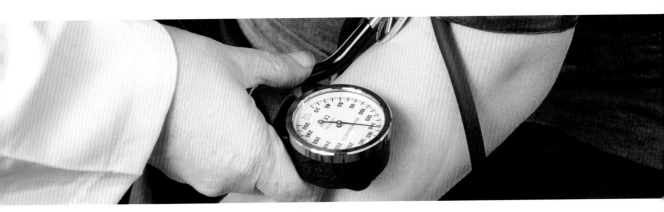

Common Liver Problems and Liver Function Test Abnormalities Seen

	Bilirubin	ALT & AST	ALP & GGT	Albumin
Acute Liver Damage e.g. infection, toxins, drugs	Normal	Greatly increased and ALT > AST	Normal	Normal
Fatty Liver Disease (alcohol related or non-alcohol related)	Normal	Slightly increased and AST > ALT (in alcohol-related injury) or ALT > AST (in non-alcohol related liver injury)	Normal or GGT slightly elevated (in alcohol-related liver injury)	Normal
Alcoholic Hepatitis	Normal	Greatly increased and AST > ALT	ALP can be increased and GGT is usually increased	Normal
Cirrhosis	Normal	Increased and AST > ALT	Normal or increased	Decreased
Gallstones	Normal or increased	Normal	Greatly increased	Normal or slightly decreased

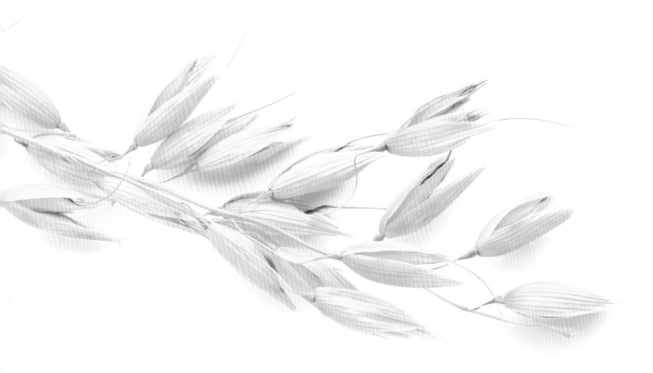

Albumin is a protein produced by the liver that is used to transport many substances such as hormones around the body. In severe liver damage the production of albumin is reduced and so this is reflected in blood testing.

Bilirubin is a breakdown product of red blood cells and is stored in the gallbladder. When there is significant gallbladder disease bilirubin can spill over into the bloodstream leading to yellowing of the skin. There is a relatively common genetic condition, however, known as Gilbert's syndrome, which causes a slight elevation in bilirubin levels from a young age. This condition is thought to be benign and of no clinical significance. Usually in this condition there are no other markers of liver damage that are elevated, distinguishing it from other causes of elevated bilirubin levels such as gallstones.

ALT stands for alanine aminotransferase and is one of the liver markers. Note that in acute liver damage its level will be higher in the blood than AST, whereas in alcoholic hepatitis and cirrhosis of the liver AST will be higher than ALT.

AST stands for aspartate aminotransferase and is another liver marker that can indicate liver cell damage. It can also be an indication of damage to our muscles or our heart.

ALP stands for alkaline phosphatase and is often elevated in liver disease caused by gallbladder or bile-duct disease such as gallstones. It can also be elevated in bone diseases.

GGT stands for Gamma-Glutamyl Transpeptidase and is often elevated in alcohol-related liver injury as well as from gallbladder/bile-duct disease.

- Ultrasound scan of the liver – if liver damage is suspected your doctor may arrange an ultrasound of your liver as well as surrounding organs such as gallbladder and pancreas. An ultrasound will assess the size of your liver to check that it isn't enlarged and will also detect fatty liver disease and other structural abnormalities.

- Other scans – if any abnormalities are detected on the ultrasound then your doctor may arrange for you to have a computed tomography (CT) scan or magnetic resonance imaging (MRI) of your liver. These provide further information about the structure of the liver.

- Biopsy – if severe liver damage is suspected, for example cirrhosis of the liver, your doctor will arrange for you to be referred to a liver specialist (known as a hepatologist or gastroenterologist) to have a liver biopsy. Very few individuals require a liver biopsy, which can be a painful procedure. In this type of testing, a small piece of liver tissue is removed and examined under the microscope in a laboratory.

Once liver damage is detected, or even if liver damage is not picked up on blood testing or other testing but you have symptoms consistent with liver damage, the best way to restore optimal liver function is to provide an environment that will allow the liver to heal.

This is the basis of Your Liver Detox Plan. But first let us look in detail at the things that may damage the liver so that we can avoid these substances and situations and prevent our liver health from deteriorating or, if deterioration has already occurred, to allow it to heal. I have called these liver assailants the 'Liver Haters'.

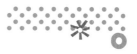

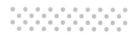

▶ ▶ ▶

LIVER
HATERS

▼▼▼▼▼▼▼▼▼▼▼▼▼▼▼▼▼▼▼▼▼▼▼▼▼▼▼▼▼▼▼▼▼
···

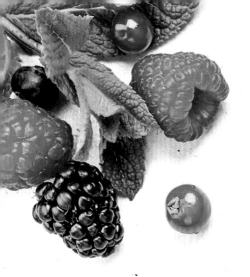

conditions is explained further in the section Your Liver Detox Plan).

When our liver is not functioning optimally due to these conditions we do not feel very well at all. In fact, the state of our liver can so significantly impact our overall health that I have seen individuals completely debilitated by their liver disease.

One patient in particular comes to mind. He was an otherwise fit gentleman of normal body weight but had found that, in recent years, he was indulging in what he called 'the good life'. Too much alcohol, caffeine and café lunches had lead to some liver damage. His main symptoms were fatigue, a bloated abdomen, itchy skin especially at night, and an offensive taste in his mouth that he described as 'metallic'. These symptoms were really starting to affect his quality of life to the point where he was taking time off work thinking he must be stressed. On blood testing his liver function markers were elevated, in particular GGT, ALT and AST. His bad cholesterol levels were slightly elevated as was his blood sugar level. When he made some necessary lifestyle adjustments, these symptoms largely resolved and all of his biochemical blood markers returned to normal.

Did you know that you can damage your liver without even knowing? There needs to be considerable damage done to your liver to result in symptoms, which might make it difficult for you to know if something is wrong. There are also a number of common, seemingly harmless substances that will damage your liver when accumulated over time. These substances can be environmental or lifestyle-related and because they can be particularly nasty in their cumulative effects on the liver I call them the 'Liver Haters'.

The damaging effects from these Liver Haters can go on to form conditions of the liver that prevent it from performing its vital functions. The most common I see in clinical practice is fatty liver disease, followed by acute liver inflammation and gallbladder disease, which I will describe (an explanation on how to reverse these

How Can Your Liver Be Damaged?

There are three main categories of Liver Haters that damage the liver. These include toxins, overload agents and micro-organisms. They are all relatively common and it may really surprise you to know how much they can harm the liver over time.

Toxins

A toxin is a substance or compound that can be stored in our body's fat deposits and so can accumulate over a lifetime, leading to a toxic load on our body as we age.

Additionally, some substances that may not be toxic to the liver in small amounts can lead to liver damage if there is a large amount of that substance present in our system that the liver has to process. An example of this is paracetamol, a common painkiller. If someone ingests too much paracetamol at once or over time, then this toxic compound accumulates in the liver and can lead to liver damage. In

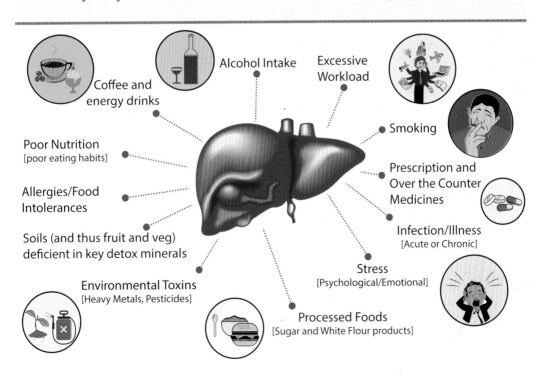

Everyday substances that can damage your liver

Coffee and energy drinks

Alcohol Intake

Excessive Workload

Smoking

Poor Nutrition
[poor eating habits]

Allergies/Food Intolerances

Prescription and Over the Counter Medicines

Infection/Illness
[Acute or Chronic]

Soils (and thus fruit and veg) deficient in key detox minerals

Stress
[Psychological/Emotional]

Environmental Toxins
[Heavy Metals, Pesticides]

Processed Foods
[Sugar and White Flour products]

extreme cases, if a very large amount of paracetamol is ingested at once (twenty or more tablets) or repeatedly over a few days (at least ten or more tablets each day), liver failure and even death can occur[2].

Along with damage to the liver itself, if the liver's detoxification processes become overloaded then the build-up of toxic chemicals can spill over into the bloodstream causing all sorts of problems. Issues such as the following can start to appear:

- Brain dysfunction and 'brain fog'

- Hormonal disruption leading to imbalance in the ratio of progesterone to oestrogen levels in the body. This can cause breast pain, menstrual issues, mood swings and has even been implicated in breast cancer development.

- Immune system irritation leading to inflammation. This can heighten allergies and allergic responses, exacerbate inflammatory diseases like arthritis, cause autoimmune diseases, swollen glands, recurrent infections and/or chronic fatigue syndrome and fibromyalgia.

Some of the toxins that we come into contact with in daily life that can damage our liver include:

- Industrial pollution

- Some pesticides, which can be residual on unwashed fruit and vegetables

- Some cleaning products

- Plastics e.g. bisphenol-A (BPA) found in some food storage containers, baby bottles and plastic toys, and plastic cutlery

- Cigarette smoke

- Recreational drugs

- Alcohol

- Heavy metals e.g. mercury, aluminium, cadmium, lead and copper

- Many artificial food additives

- Certain medications such as paracetamol, and certain antibiotics and anti-fungal medications

Overload Agents – sugar, excess carbs, unhealthy fats and red meat

It is very easy to overindulge in today's society where food is plentiful. This can easily overload the liver's ability to breakdown and process food nutrients in addition to the other common substances in our diet such as caffeine and alcohol.

Along with caffeine and alcohol, those other substances, which I collectively call the 'Overload Agents', are:

- **Fructose** – a type of sugar found in fruit, processed foods and cane sugar

- **Refined carbohydrates** – foods made with white flours, such as cakes, biscuits, pastries and muffins. Refined carbohydrates are essentially converted to pure sugar by the body anyway. Even gluten-free foods aren't that healthy if made with certain types of flours such as white rice flour.

- **Unhealthy fats** – including trans fats found in some processed foods such as cakes and biscuits as well as excessive amounts of saturated fats found in animal products.

- **Iron-rich foods** – including excessive red meat and supplements containing iron. These are only potentially harmful if the liver is already inflamed due to liver disease as an inflamed liver will store extra iron. Too much iron in the liver can lead to liver cell damage. You can check your liver iron stores by a simple blood test known as a ferritin level as arranged by your local doctor. If this is higher than 200ng/mL for men or 150ng/mL for women then excessive red meat intake and iron supplements need to be avoided.

Many patients with an unhealthy liver, who I have seen in clinical practice, do not eat too many calories. Quite the opposite – they are either hardly eating (which poses its own metabolic issues by causing the body to go into a state where it stores more body fat) or they are eating the wrong types of calories (that is, calories from the wrong types of fats and sugars and that place a heavy burden on the liver). As already explained, our liver is the fat-and-sugar processing plant of the body. If we eat the wrong types of fats and sugars consistently this essentially overburdens the liver and leads to it being unable to perform its metabolic functions. The result is a reduced fat-burning and sugar-burning ability, fatty liver disease and weight gain around the middle. You will feel tired, sluggish and frumpy.

The liver also takes the excess dietary fat that you are eating and converts this into cholesterol, which in turn makes bile. Bile is pumped out of your body via the intestines if your diet is high in fibre. So essentially if your liver is healthy and your gallbladder works your body will be able to eliminate the excess fat you are eating. The liver also produces proteins, 'lipoproteins', which are a form of cholesterol. These proteins help to transport fat around the bloodstream. If you are eating too much of the wrong types of fats you will develop an imbalance in the different lipoproteins:

You will have an increase in your 'low-density lipoprotein (LDL)' (unhealthy cholesterol) which sacrifices the production of your 'high-density lipoprotein (HDL)' (healthy cholesterol). LDL can lead to clogged arteries and cardiovascular disease whereas HDL protects you from this.

You may have also heard of triglycerides, which are a particularly harmful form of cholesterol. Triglycerides are made by the liver when too many bad fats (trans fats and saturated fats) are eaten as well as too much sugar. A deficiency in essential fatty acids can also increase triglyceride levels.

Some people do have a genetic predisposition to a high level of HDL being produced by their liver, which offers them more protection from heart disease (to a point, of course, as genetics can be overridden by a poor diet and lifestyle), but the rest of us rely heavily on our liver to produce LDL and HDL in balance. When LDL and HDL levels become imbalanced in favour of LDL

production we have a problem! The solution is not always to go on cholesterol-lowering medications but, rather, to first address our lifestyles and clean up our livers! The slippery slope of starting medication is that there is often a false sense of security that you are 'covered' from heart disease. But cholesterol is only one component of cardiovascular health.

There are other factors that stem from an unhealthy body and an unhealthy liver that can lead to cardiovascular disease, such as high blood pressure and increased total body inflammation from carrying too much weight around our mid-sections and from our toxic lifestyles. These also are corrected when we look after our health, which starts with our liver health. This is what Your Liver Detox Plan specifically addresses. It will help to reverse high bad cholesterol levels and reduce body fat stores.

Micro-Organisms – viruses, bacteria in food poisoning

Certain organisms present in our environment can damage the liver by either directly attacking the body or via the chemicals the organisms produce as they die off. The nastiest organisms that can cause liver damage include:

- Blood-borne Hepatitis viruses – Hepatitis C and B (transmitted by blood and other body fluids)

- Food-borne Hepatitis viruses – Hepatitis A and E (transmitted via contaminated food)

- Food-borne bacteria – E.coli, salmonella, campylobacter. These are found in contaminated food such as undercooked chicken and can cause the symptoms of food poisoning. Avoid food poisoning by properly preparing and cooking raw meats, especially chicken.

- HIV

- Malaria

- Tuberculosis

- Epstein-Barr Virus (EBV) and Cytomegalovirus (CMV) – EBV causes glandular fever.

It is also believed that an imbalance in the gut flora that live normally in our digestive system can cause liver health issues through the toxins these organisms produce as part of their metabolic processes. One such organism is clostridium difficile, an overgrowth caused by long-term antibiotic use[3]. Other organisms implicated in liver damage include streptococcus and enterococcus. These are also thought to be responsible for the creation of food intolerance symptoms such as bloating and abdominal pain.

It is important to restore proper gut flora balance in order to improve overall health and wellbeing as well as liver health. How to do this will be explained a little later on.

Other Conditions

Note that there are some inherited diseases that can cause liver damage including those that lead to copper and iron accumulation, known as Wilson's disease and hereditary haemochromatosis, respectively. Luckily these conditions are able to be picked up during blood testing. If you have a family history of liver disease it is worth mentioning this to your doctor who can run some simple testing to rule these conditions out.

Diseases that cause damage to the intestinal lining and therefore allow large, unprocessed molecules through the intestinal wall into the bloodstream can also overwhelm the liver. These conditions include Crohn's disease, ulcerative colitis, coeliac disease, and to some degree issues of food intolerance such as gluten intolerance (non-coeliac), lactose intolerance and food-chemical intolerance. It is important to address these issues in order to heal and support your liver function as well as digestive health in order to feel better. For an explanation of food intolerances and treatment approaches refer to the relevant chapters in my book *Healthy Habits: 52 Ways to Better Health*.

Common Conditions of the Liver

Liver damage resulting from the conditions listed below can develop into a serious liver problem if not kept in check relatively early and quickly. These conditions often go unrecognised as they may initially not cause any obvious symptoms.

The most common liver conditions include:

- **Fatty Liver Disease** – this is the most common cause of liver disease in Western countries[4]. Fat accumulates inside liver cells, causing cell enlargement and sometimes cell damage and impairment of liver function. In fatty liver disease the liver becomes enlarged, causing discomfort on the upper right side of the abdomen. Fatty liver can occur if we are carrying too much weight for our frame, have diabetes, have an inflamed liver due to toxin overload, or because we have been consuming too much fructose, refined carbohydrates, processed fats and/or alcohol.

- **Metabolic Syndrome** – related to fatty liver disease but also includes a cluster of health issues including high blood pressure, elevated bad cholesterol levels, low good cholesterol levels, impaired glucose tolerance (which can lead to type 2 diabetes), and carrying a significant amount of weight around your mid-section. Not everyone who develops fatty liver disease will have metabolic syndrome but most of those with metabolic syndrome will have a level of fatty liver disease[5]. This is a condition to be taken seriously with the main cause of death long-term being from heart disease. To reverse this condition lifestyle changes need to be implemented, including those mentioned in this book.

- **Hepatitis** – this is a condition caused by inflammation of the liver leading to damage and impaired function. It may be caused by fatty liver disease, alcohol damage and damage from micro-organisms (the most common being hepatitis C and B) among other causes.

If hepatitis is not treated and reversed it can develop into cirrhosis of the liver.

- Cirrhosis of the Liver – is the end-result of many liver conditions and involves severe scarring of the liver (with liver nodule formation). It is associated with a progressive decline in liver function and can result in liver failure as well as liver cancer.

- Acute Liver Inflammation – this is when the liver cells become acutely inflamed from a recent, and usually short-lived, injury. The most common cause of acute liver inflammation is an adverse reaction to medication, but it may also occur due to another type of infection such as Epstein-Barr Virus (glandular fever). If liver enzyme markers in a recent blood test are elevated then this might be the reason.

- Gallbladder Disease or Bile-Duct Disease – gallbladder disease or bile-duct disease can occur when gallstones form and lodge in the bile ducts 'the plumbing system' of the liver, causing inflammation, pain and damage. Gallbladder disease is relatively common and may affect as many as 1 in 5 women and 1 in 10 men in Australia[6].

The main cause of this disease is thought to be consumption of too much unhealthy dietary fat and/or carbohydrates, which are turned into bad cholesterol by the liver. The liver will in turn attempt to remove this cholesterol through bile, which is deposited into the small intestine and eventually moved out of the body. Bile then becomes saturated with bad cholesterol and the result is hard gallstones made of solidified cholesterol. Gallbladder disease can cause severe upper abdominal pain that may radiate into the back and/or into the right shoulder. It is accompanied by nausea and vomiting and an intolerance to fatty foods.

Your Guide to Liver Hating Foods

This guide highlights some bad food for the liver as well as some foods that should be eaten in moderation.

Proteins

These sources of protein should be eaten in moderation so as not to overload the liver:

- Beef

- Pork

- Lamb

- Sausages

- Bacon or ham

- Shellfish including prawns, shellfish, oysters, mussels or crab

- Veal

- Fish higher in mercury content, such as shark, orange roughy, swordfish and ling

- Limit canned tuna to 2-3 serves per week

- Smoked or cured fish e.g. smoked salmon (higher in nitrates, which are to be avoided)

- Deli meats (roast and slice your own chicken or turkey for lunches)

Beans and Legumes

Beans and Legumes are great for overall health, but try to choose unsalted varieties. Avoid:

- Flavoured or salted canned beans. If possible, prepare your own by soaking overnight and either boiling or pressure cooking. If not possible, choose unsalted canned varieties that contain no preservatives or additives.

Starches and Grains

These starches and grains should be consumed in moderation:

- Wheat products (including bread, pasta, crackers, cakes, pastries, biscuits, muesli bars or breakfast cereals)

- Rye

- Barley

- Spelt

- Couscous

- Triticale

- Chips (all types)

Vegetables

Vegetables are fabulous for overall health, but fresh is always best. Avoid:

- Pickled

- Tinned

- Frozen

Fruit

Fruit is great in moderation, but avoid fruit that has been dried or candied as it is high in sugar. Avoid:

- Canned

- Dried

- Candied or crystallised

- Concentrated fruit juice

Dairy
Avoid:

- Cheese (eat in moderation)
- Cream
- Ice-cream
- Sweetened yoghurts
- Custard

Nuts and seeds
Avoid:

- Peanuts
- Roasted or salted nuts
- Candied or chocolate-covered nuts

Oils

- Butter
- Canola oil
- Duck fat
- Ghee
- Margerine
- Peanut oil
- Vegetable oil

Herbs and Spices, Dressings and Condiments
Avoid:

- Sugar
- Salt
- Sweetened spices such as sweetened cinnamon
- Artificial sweeteners

Drinks
Avoid:

- Alcohol
- Soft drinks
- Fruit drinks
- Coffee and tea (except herbal)
- Reconstituted juice

As explained in this chapter, although there are quite a few substances that can overwhelm and damage the liver, there is hope! Following the principles outlined in the Detox Plan will help to safeguard your liver from damage. Keep in mind that some factors, such as exposure to environmental toxins, will be beyond your control and may compromise your liver health. Ultimately, though, the balance of responsibility to protect your liver is in your hands and *is* achievable if you choose to follow the suggested guidelines in this book and, in particular, in the next two chapters.

The next chapter looks at 'Liver Lovers' and how to look after your liver day to day.

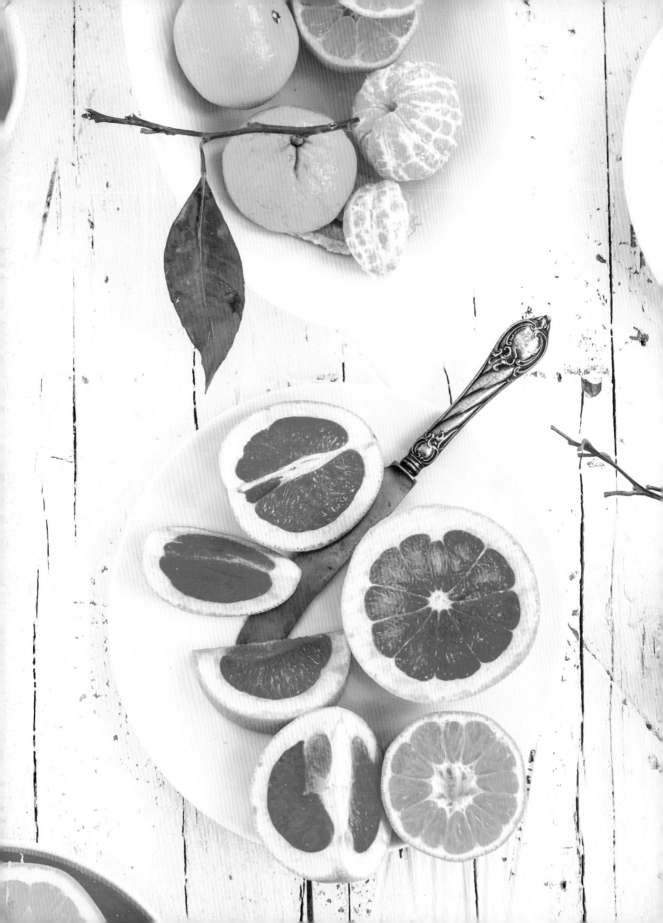

►►►

LIVER
LOVERS

▼▼▼▼▼▼▼▼▼▼▼▼▼▼▼▼▼▼▼▼▼▼▼▼▼▼▼▼▼
···

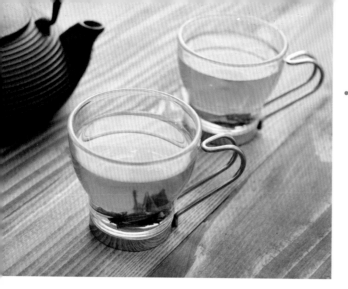

The secret to great health is to be a lover and not a hater – a Liver Lover, that is! Our liver really is the health gateway to the rest of our body. If we can maintain our liver health by following the 'liver loving' suggestions below then good health will be our reward.

Strategies to support and maintain liver health can be broken down into several categories – liver loving foods, lifestyles, and supportive supplements.

Liver Loving Foods

The Liver Loving Foods are those that support liver function and, in particular, liver detoxification pathways. They boost liver function and with it liver health. These foods include:

- Vegetables from the 'brassica' family – broccoli, kale, cauliflower, Brussels sprouts and cabbage. The protective effect of the brassicas on the liver is due to their high content of glucosinolates. Once these vegetables are chewed and digested, glucosinolates are converted into two types of highly reactive compounds, which work together as powerful stimulants for the liver's detoxification pathways. Eating a serve of these types of vegetables regularly (I usually advise at least three times per week) will help give your liver a boost. Foods that are high in sulphur also help promote liver detoxification. This includes onions and garlic. Vegetables containing dark pigments can also help with liver health. These include pumpkins, red cabbage, carrots, capsicums and beetroot.

- Fruits containing ellagic acid such as raspberries and red grapes, and citrus fruits such as oranges and lemons.

- Herbs and spices including rosemary, fennel, celery seed, cumin, dill and turmeric. Dandelion has been shown to increase bile output and thereby is thought to potentially aid liver detoxification[7].

- Proteins – the liver needs quality proteins to function optimally. Good protein sources include lean meats, legumes, beans, and wholegrains such as quinoa, buckwheat and millet.

- Green tea – has also been shown to support liver detoxification[8]. Remember, though, that green tea contains caffeine so do avoid excessive amounts.

Incorporating these foods regularly in your diet will steer you towards a Liver Loving Lifestyle, which supports good liver health rather than deteriorates it.

Liver Loving Lifestyles

A lifestyle that favours liver health is one based on moderation. As with anything, a total avoidance of any particular substance can lead to cravings and bingeing. A better approach is to include those things that you just can't give up in small amounts. The exception, of course, being cigarette smoking and illicit drug use. Those substances are too harmful to the body to have in any amount. Smoking is extremely challenging to give up due to its addictive element. Do seek help and guidance from your local doctor, who can offer the best quitting strategy for you.

80:20 Rule

When it comes to food think 80:20. Eighty per cent of your diet should be made up of fresh, unprocessed foods such as wholegrains, fruits and vegetables, nuts and seeds, eggs and lean meats. The other twenty per cent of you diet can be all the other things you love to eat but in moderation. This includes sweets, cheeses and processed foods.

Listen to Your Hunger Cues

Many of us overeat and therefore place an extra load on our livers. This can easily lead to liver disease without us ever actually eating anything 'bad'. The result is that we end up with poor health. Learn to listen to your hunger cues and try not to allow yourself to become ravenously hungry. This will help to prevent gorging, which can happen when you try to raise blood sugar levels that have dropped.

Similarly, avoid eating when you are not hungry. We can eat for a variety of reasons with hunger usually being the least obvious. Sometimes we eat because we are tired, bored, stressed, angry, lonely, feeling low or because we are procrastinating. Learn to recognise when you are eating as a result of your emotions rather than actual hunger and try to reduce the times that you eat when you are not hungry.

Hydrate Well

One of the easiest things you can do to love your liver is to drink plenty of water. Ideally aim for filtered water and drink at least 2 litres per day, more if it is hot or if you are doing heavy exercise and sweating a lot. To check you are drinking enough water look at the colour of your urine; it should be light straw-coloured or clear. The exception of course being if you are taking B vitamins or vitamin C, which can discolour your urine for a few hours afterwards. Keep in mind that liquid in the form of tea, coffee, alcohol, soft drinks, juice and ice blocks does not count. Herbal teas, which do not contain caffeine can be counted as a cup of water.

Eat Healthy Fats

There are three types of fat in our diet – good, bad and ugly. Bad and ugly fats can clog our arteries and lead to liver disease if eaten in excess. They are 'unhealthy fats'. Good fats or 'healthy fats', on the other hand, are beneficial to our health. Many of us are 'fat-phobic' due to the legacy of our previous understanding of nutrition. We now realise that you need to have some fat in your diet[9]. If you completely eliminate fats from your diet you may become essential fatty acid deficient; the symptoms of which include dry and itchy skin, eczema, joint pain, low mood, reduced immunity, hair loss and mild memory loss. Fats also increase the feeling of fullness when you eat and so you are less likely to overeat if there

is some fat in your meal. Like anything, however, you can have too much of a good thing and so moderation is key.

Bad fats are saturated and damaged fats. Saturated fats are found in fatty cuts of meat and dairy products such as milk, yoghurt, cheese and chocolate. Too much of this type of fat can raise bad cholesterol levels in the blood, which is thought to lead to heart disease as well as fatty liver disease[10]. 'Damaged fats' are fats that have been converted to toxic compounds by the cooking process. There are certain oils that should not be used for cooking due to their low smoke point, which means that when they are heated in cooking they convert to toxic and potentially harmful fats. For this reason, frying foods at high temperatures should be avoided. Avoid deep-fried foods and instead choose to lightly stir-fry your foods or consider frying in water, first, as they do in Asian cooking, adding a small amount of oil, such as sesame oil, in later for flavour. Try coconut oil, macadamia oil, sunflower, grapeseed and rice bran oils for stir-fry dishes. These oils have a higher smoke point.

Ugly fats are found in processed foods and are called 'trans fats'. Trans fats are manmade and are included in processed foods to increase their shelf life. The issue with trans fats is that they are foreign to the body and can cause inflammation, liver disease, clogged arteries and weight gain. Avoid the ugly trans fats in your diet – there is simply no place for them. Do read labels and make sure that the products you are buying do not include trans fats, which are often named 'shortening' or 'partially hydrogenated vegetable oil' on the ingredients list. Most biscuits, crackers, pie crusts, pizza dough, cakes, muffins, pastries, instant soup mixes, stocks, chicken nuggets, fish fingers, margarine, microwavable popcorn, chips and instant noodles contain this ingredient unless specified as containing 'no trans fats' on the packaging.

The good fats are the polyunsaturated fats (these include the omega-3 and -6 essential fatty acids) and monounsaturated fats. Eating foods rich in monounsaturated and polyunsaturated fat can improve blood cholesterol levels and lower your risk of heart disease. These fats may also benefit insulin levels and control blood sugar, which can be especially helpful if you have type 2 diabetes. These good fats include:

Monounsaturated fat
Avocados
Olives
Nuts (almonds, peanuts, macadamia nuts, hazelnuts, pecans, cashews)
Natural peanut butter (containing just peanuts and salt)
Polyunsaturated fat (including omega-3 and -6 fats)
Walnuts
Sunflower seeds, sesame seeds, safflower seeds and pumpkin seeds
Flaxseed (linseeds)
Evening primrose oil
Lecithin
Spirulina
Fatty fish (salmon, tuna, mackerel, herring, trout, sardines)
Non-genetically modified sources of soy milk and tofu

Just a word on omega-3 fatty essential acids, which is a type of polyunsaturated fat. It is often deficient in Western diets, which contributes to a lot of the disease that we see in clinical practice[11]. Omega-3 fatty acids have been found to:

- Play a vital role in cognitive function (memory, problem-solving abilities etc.)

- Prevent and reduce the symptoms of depression, ADHD and bipolar disorder

- Protect against memory loss and dementia

- Reduce the risk of heart disease, stroke and cancer

- Ease arthritis, joint pain and inflammatory skin conditions

- Support a healthy pregnancy

- Help you battle fatigue, sharpen your memory and balance your mood

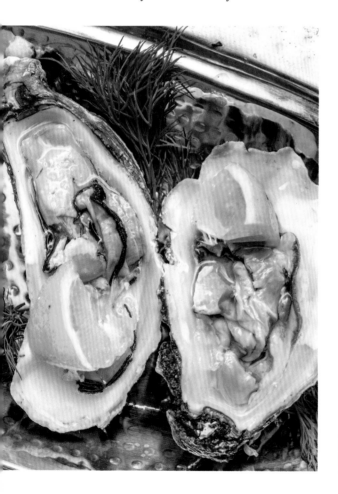

We need to have omega-6 and -3 essential fatty acids (often referred to as omega-3 and -6 fats) in balance, as with most things in our diet. Omega-6 essential fatty acid, also a type of polyunsaturated fat, is found in plenty of the foods that we would eat day-to-day, whereas omega-3 fats are found in more specific foods and so can be easily missed in our diet. The best sources of omega-3 fats are listed below.

Good Fats

Fish: the best source of omega-3s
Salmon (especially wild-caught king and sockeye)
Herring
Mackerel
Anchovies
Oysters
Sardines
Pole and line-caught tuna
Lake trout
Vegetarian sources of omega-3s
Algae such as seaweed
Fish oil or algae supplements
Walnuts
Flaxseed
Brussels sprouts
Kale
Spinach
Parsley

Alcohol

As for alcohol, many of us overindulge and drink way too much. The recommended safe limit for health is no more than one standard drink per day for women with two alcohol-free days per week, and no more than two standard drinks per day for men also with two alcohol-free days per week[12]. Ideally the two alcohol-free days should be consecutive to give the liver a rest. Keep in mind that a standard drink is equivalent to 100MLs of wine (half a standard wine glass), 1 mid-strength beer, or 30MLs of spirits (a nip). So a bottle of wine should last a person around four to seven nights.

Caffeine

Caffeine is another favourite indulgence and for some a necessity! There are some benefits to caffeine but you can have too much. Up to 200mg (about 3–4 cups of instant coffee or tea) of caffeine in adults can stimulate liver function, which can be a good thing to aid metabolism and detoxification[13, 14]. Amounts of caffeine consumed above this, however, can cause some liver damage, so cut down if you are consuming too much caffeine. You can replace your coffee with a decaffeinated variety but be sure that the caffeine-removal process is natural, without the use of chemicals. Look for organic and water-filtered brands (usually available at health food stores).

Your Guide to Liver Loving Foods

Here is a specific list of foods that love your liver:

Protein

- ✓ Chicken
- ✓ Eggs
- ✓ Fresh fish (except those on the avoid list)
- ✓ Calamari
- ✓ Tempeh or tofu
- ✓ Turkey
- ✓ Protein powder supplements (optional) such as brown rice protein or pea protein. These contain very little carbohydrates and are mostly protein. Ideally avoid whey protein which can cause digestion issues in some individuals. A serve is one heaped tablespoon.

Beans and Legumes

- ✓ Broad beans
- ✓ Borlotti beans
- ✓ Butter beans
- ✓ Kidney Beans
- ✓ Chickpeas
- ✓ Lima beans
- ✓ Pinto beans
- ✓ Black beans
- ✓ Navy beans
- ✓ Split peas
- ✓ Lentils
- ✓ Adzuki beans
- ✓ Alfalfa sprouts

Starches and Grains

- ✓ Brown or wild rice
- ✓ Buckwheat
- ✓ Millet
- ✓ Quinoa
- ✓ Amaranth
- ✓ Traditional or steel cut oats (not instant)
- ✓ Corn

- ✓ Gluten-free flours made from the above
- ✓ Gluten-free rice or corn cakes or crackers (unflavoured)
- ✓ Almond or hazelnut meals
- ✓ Coconut flour

Vegetables

- ✓ All vegetables (except potato)
- ✓ All salad greens
- ✓ Fermented vegetables including sauerkraut or kimchi (these can be fermented at home or store-bought as organic varieties)

Fruits

- ✓ All fresh fruit (this includes avocados, but limit to ¼ avocado per day)
- ✓ Frozen berries (fresh is best but often expensive)

Dairy

- ✓ Goat's or sheep's milk (often easier to digest)
- ✓ Cow's milk (unhomogenised and/or A2, which is easier to digest and is available from most supermarkets)

- ✓ Plain unsweetened yoghurt

Nuts and Seeds

- ✓ Almonds (around 20 almonds)
- ✓ Brazil nuts (limit to 5 per day)
- ✓ Chia seeds
- ✓ Coconut
- ✓ Hazelnuts
- ✓ Linseeds/flaxseeds
- ✓ Macadamia nuts
- ✓ Pecans
- ✓ Pepitas
- ✓ Pine nuts
- ✓ Sesame seeds
- ✓ Sunflower seeds
- ✓ Walnuts

Oils

- ✓ Olive oil (for dressings only, not cooking)
- ✓ Macadamia oil
- ✓ Flaxseed (linseed) oil
- ✓ Rice bran oil
- ✓ Sesame oil
- ✓ Grapeseed oil
- ✓ Walnut oil
- ✓ Coconut oil
- ✓ Avocado oil

Herbs and Spices, Dressings and Condiments

- ✓ Lemon juice
- ✓ Apple cider vinegar
- ✓ Red or white wine vinegar
- ✓ Organic tamari
- ✓ Balsamic vinegar (limit to 1-2 tsps per day due to sugar content)

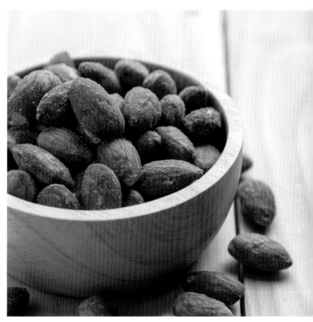

✓ Mustard

✓ Tahini

✓ Stevia or xylitol

✓ Honey (limit to 1-2 tsps per day)

✓ Rice bran or malt syrup (limit to 1-2 tsps per day)

Drinks

✓ Still or sparking water

✓ Non-caffeinated herbal teas such as dandelion, Tulsi tear, or herbal infusions (no added sugar)

✓ Green tea or Oolong tea (limit to 2-3 cups per day)

✓ Fresh vegetable juices

Exercise

Lastly, exercise has been shown to aid liver function by improving the body's usage of fats and glucose. Exercise is an important part of a Liver Loving Lifestyle and ideally needs to be included in your weekly routine – at least thirty minutes most days of the week. If you are not used to exercising, build up your exercise time slowly. If you find you just do not have the time to exercise, consider incorporating short bursts of activity in ten-minute blocks throughout the day such as before work, in your lunch break or/and after work. This has been shown to be just as effective as a full thirty-minute stretch of exercise.

Stress Less

It is understood that high levels of emotional stress (e.g from untreated depression and anxiety, from relationship tensions, or from long-held negative beliefs) and/or physical stress (e.g. from staying up late at night, from working long hours, from overtraining with exercise, and from not resting) can all place a load on the body and, in turn, the liver. This is due to toxic chemicals created in the body as a result of stress, all of which lead to increased total body inflammation[15]. It is not unusual for me to see elevated liver markers in professional athletes and signs of body inflammation just from the training load they place themselves under, even though they are obviously very healthy. These individuals require extra nutrients to offset the load their training places on their bodies and liver. They often also require extra rest to allow their bodies to effectively detox and recover.

For the rest of us, the best way to offset the impact of stress on the body is to learn to stress a little less. Taking time to deal with negative emotions – either through personal reflection or counselling – can have a profound effect on the body's ability to heal. Find the time to rest and recover by sleeping enough hours at night, resting on the weekends and having some time for 'play' rather than just all work. Utilise gentle exercise such as walking, yoga, Pilates and other forms of gentle physical activity to dissipate tension. Do whatever you need to do to reduce the amount of stress in your life. If that's simply not possible, try to build your internal physical and emotional resilience to the amount of stress in your life by incorporating the above strategies in small but significant ways.

To further boost a lifestyle that is promoting liver health there are some supplements that you can take. Keep in mind these do not replace a healthy diet but, rather, add to it.

Living-Loving Supplements

The supplements listed here are considered supportive of liver function and may aid and even speed up your liver's recovery[16]. For a list of specific supplements to suit your liver health refer to *Step Four – Choose Liver Supplements Wisely* in the section Your Liver Detox Plan.

Herbs	Schizandra, St John's wort, rosemary, milk thistle, turmeric, dandelion root
Antioxidant	Coenzyme Q10, bioflavonoids, alpha lipoic acid
Vitamins	The antioxidant vitamins A, C and E as well as thiamin (B1), niacin (B3), pyridoxine (B6), B12, and folic acid
Minerals	Zinc, selenium, manganese, magnesium
Amino Acids	Cysteine, glutathione, L-glycine, L.-glutamine, taurine and methylation cofactors. Because glutathione is poorly absorbed from the digestive tract it is often given as N-acetyl cysteine (NAC)

Just a word about starting any new supplements – always consult your doctor to ensure correct dosage and possible interactions with any other medicines you may be taking.

Now that we have covered generally how to love your liver, we are ready to embark upon the next section of this book with the Liver Detox Plan, which will put together all of these Liver Loving principles in an easy-to-follow format.

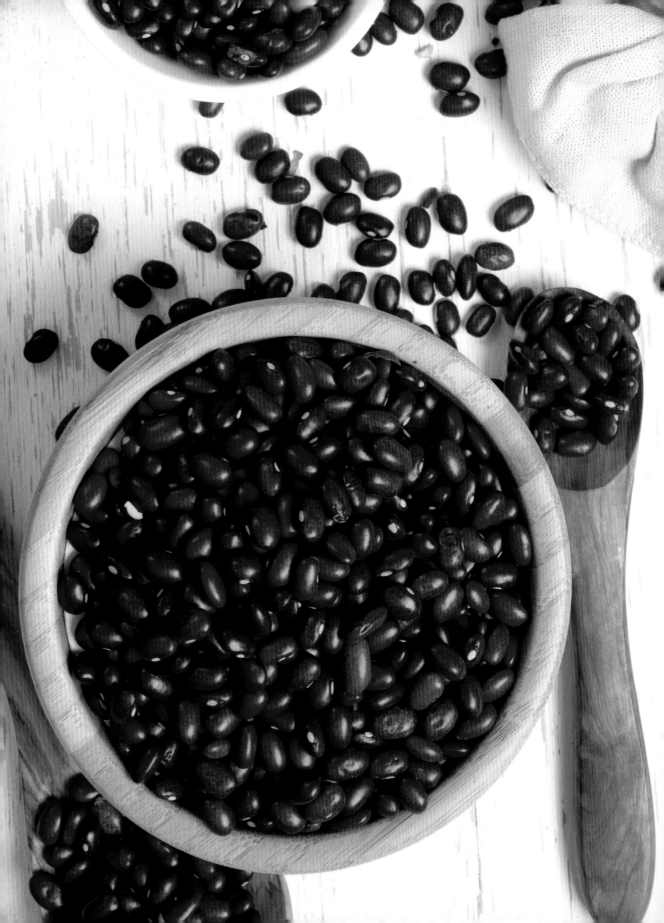

▶ ▶ ▶

YOUR
LIVER
DETOX
PLAN

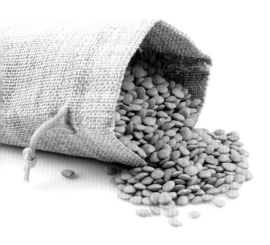

The word detox is a buzz-word these days. It's often attached to marketing a particular product, supplement or diet that claims to clear out the liver and return liver function to normal. But do these detoxes actually work and what does the word 'detox' mean.

Detox often refers to 'detoxifying' the liver by removing any build-up of toxins or substances that can overload it, such as those we have already discussed in the chapter on 'Liver Haters', reducing the liver's ability to function normally. The issue with relying on one particular product, supplement or strict diet to detoxify the liver is that this creates a reliance on these to be able to return your liver to good health. In reality, the liver is an amazing regenerative organ. It is able to regenerate itself almost completely even when significant damage is present. The exception of course being cirrhosis,

which is when the liver tissue has been so scarred by chronic damage that a portion of the liver becomes non-functional. Saying that, even in cirrhosis of the liver, the remaining healthy liver tissue is able to take over liver functioning if given the right environment.

So how do you *really* detox your liver? The key is to provide your liver with a healing environment. That is, one that is free of ongoing insult, and one that is permissive to allow natural liver regeneration and repair to take place in order to return optimal liver functioning. This essentially means that no particular product or strict diet is the solution but, rather, a shift in lifestyle. Another problem with relying on a strict diet is that it is often not sustainable. As soon as you stop following the diet and return to your usual lifestyle you will find the same problems occurring with your liver.

To simplify the process of detoxification I find the best strategy is to follow this Detox. I call this Your Liver Detox Plan and it includes preparing for your detox, eliminating toxins, following the 7-Day Liver Detox Diet and using the menu-plan and recipes included in this book as a guide, choosing liver supplements wisely, supporting your Detox and maintaining your healthy liver. This plan is meant to be specific to you and so, where possible, I have included options that may suit your individual needs depending on your current individual liver health, which was determined by your Liver Health Score, and what your individual food and lifestyle preferences may be. I have also included alternatives in the Detox recipes, and all the ingredients should be found in most local supermarkets and food produce stores. Following Your Liver Detox Plan will result in the return of your liver health and overall health and wellbeing. Keep in mind that this is a process and recovery won't happen overnight. But stay the course and see the process through – I promise you won't regret it! Are you ready to feel better than you've ever felt? Here is Your Liver Detox Plan.

Step One – Prepare for Your Detox

A fundamental step in detoxing your liver is preparation. As they say, failing to prepare is preparing to fail. Preparation in this process requires you to consider a few key questions:

Is this the right time? Consider if your life is currently permitting you to be able to change. Is there just too much going on at the moment to be able to

concentrate on your health? Do you need to wait for a better time? Of course, if you keep procrastinating and putting your health last then now *is* the time to make some changes. If you know, however, that your life is just a bit busy and chaotic at the moment but will quieten down and allow you to focus on your liver health in the near future, then wait. You are more likely to be successful if you have given yourself the time to really focus on fulfilling this process in its entirety rather than having to stop and restart.

Am I truly ready to change? Much of the time we want to change but we aren't truly ready to change. Old thinking patterns could be holding us back or something in our environment may keep triggering old behaviours. The typical triggers are stress, being overtired from too much responsibility or activities, or a low level of motivation, confidence or belief in yourself that you have what it takes to change. To increase your motivation, consider writing down your reasons for change. If you have a strong enough reason or 'why' then this may help you. As for increasing your confidence, consider times when you have been successful at changing a certain behavior, even if it was a small behavior such as making your bed each morning or flossing your teeth twice a day. Use this as a reminder that you do have amazing personal strength and ability. Recognising your strengths will boost your ability to take control of your life and your health. For more on staying motivated to change refer to my first book, *Healthy Habits: 52 Ways to Better Health*.

Have I counted the cost of change?

Any time we change it's going to cost us something. It may cost you financially, perhaps having to spend a bit more money on good-quality food, or having to work less so that you can focus on your health. Or it may cost you some 'fun' by, perhaps, changing the pattern of alcohol drinking that you are used to. It may also cost others around you. It may cost your partner and friends that they no longer have a drinking or smoking buddy. You will also be surprised that when you start changing your behaviours others may feel threatened, confused or intimidated by the changes. They may try and pull you back to your old behaviours or dismiss your attempts to change by saying that people 'never really change'. Keep focussed on why it is you need to change and try to be a great role model for others. Sooner or later they will see how healthy you have become and may even join you in changing their own behaviours.

If you answered yes to the above three questions and you feel you are ready to embark on Your Liver Detox, then the next step in preparation is to clear out the pantry and fill it only with those items that are on the 'Liver-Friendly Shopping List' found at the back of this book. This might seem harsh, but if temptations are present you are more likely to succumb, even if you are the most strong-willed person. You are human, after all. Just when you are going well and you are starting to feel great, you will inevitably have a bad day at work or with the kids or with your partner and all of a sudden the chocolate bar, packet of chips, cheese and crackers or red wine will beckon you for just one bite or sip. Of course that's when you will likely have ten more bites or sips and before long feel like giving up on your detox and starting again next week. So the best approach to avoid temptation is to not have your temptations in the house.

This approach might seem mean to the other family members but in the end they want to see you healthy and happy and if you explain to them why you need to clear the pantry out I'm sure they will oblige. It will be a good thing for their health too! Explain that they are still allowed to make their own choices and if they want a 'treat' then they will just have to buy and eat those things outside of the home. Of course this is tricky with small children. If you still need to have snack foods for the kids in the home, keep these in sealed containers labelled 'for the kids only' and keep out of sight at the back of the fridge or cupboard. Even better is to find healthier alternatives for the kids to enjoy too and that way their health can benefit just as much as your health will by making positive changes for the whole family.

There is a time in any change process where you will 'relapse' and go back to your old behaviours. This is a normal part of change and may occur just once in the change process or multiple times depending on what your usual triggers are for the relapse and if these triggers are still present in your life. Do keep this in mind and don't beat yourself up. In the end, it's not whether you do this process perfectly but rather that you are making progress that matters. Get back on track by remembering why it is you want and need to change and why it is important. If you need help to change your lifestyle then do seek help from a health professional who may be able to assist you through the process.

Lastly, when preparing for a detox we need to remove any mental barriers. I think of these as supposed truths about what we have to do in order to truly be healthy. These truths are usually myths and they need to be discounted as they can prevent us from even starting because we fear the worst. Below are the most common myths relating to liver detoxing that I hear in clinical practice and that act as barriers to change.

Myth #1 – I will need to become vegan

Although there are some health benefits to eating more plant-based foods in your diet, you do not need to become vegan in order to have a healthy liver. However, most of us do eat way too much red meat and usually in preference to salad and vegetables. This can lead to health challenges such as an increased risk of bowel cancer.

Many people believe, too, that they will become anaemic if they don't eat red meat daily. In reality there are many regular meat eaters who are anaemic. This could be due to heavy menstrual blood loss, for instance, or because of regular overtraining with exercise. Likewise, there are many vegetarians who are *not* anaemic. Red meat can, however, be included in a healthy diet in moderation; that being two to three times per week. Although the 7-Day Liver Detox Diet does include red meat you will notice that it appears on the menu in the recommended moderate amount. This may be difficult for many people who are used to eating red meat every day. Try substituting red meat in your diet for the alternatives mentioned in the 7-Day Liver Detox Diet and you may just find that you acquire a taste for them.

Myth #2 – I will need to give up alcohol

Although the 7-Day Liver Detox Diet does not include alcohol (in order to give your liver a rest from having to process this toxin), this does not mean that you have to give up alcohol forever. Once your liver is healed you can go back to including it in your diet as long as you do so in moderation. Of course there will be the occasional function or special event where you may drink more than what is recommended for liver health but this should hopefully be the odd occasion not the weekly norm.

Myth #3 – I will need to give up sugar and carbs

In order to have a healthy liver you do not need to give up sugar completely. Be aware, however, that sugar is found in so many foods in our diet today, causing us to crave it more and more. This can be a real problem and can quickly overload the liver if we are consuming too much sugar.

By following the 7-Day Liver Detox Diet, which is low in sugar, you will find that your taste buds will adjust to wanting less sugar in general. This will make it easier to avoid sugary foods and you may find that when you do eat something sugary it will be too sweet for you to finish it.

As for carbohydrates, these can be consumed in excess easily in our diet and overload the liver because they are converted into sugar in the body. Although we don't need to give up carbohydrates altogether, we will need to cut down. The 7-Day Liver Detox Diet contains a balanced amount of carbohydrates so as not to overload the liver.

Myth #4 – I will need to lose a huge amount of weight

If you are very overweight, you may feel that you need to lose a large amount of body fat in order to be healthy. Although you may feel more comfortable losing this weight, you only need to lose a small amount to significantly impact your liver health. In fact, studies have indicated that losing around five to ten per cent of your body weight is usually all that is required to improve your overall health including liver health[17]. For example, if you weigh 100kg, losing just 5-10kg would be enough to improve your liver health significantly.

This would also be the amount of weight loss required to improve blood pressure, blood sugar levels, and boost sex hormones (and improve libido). Following the 7-Day Liver Detox Diet will see you lose around 0.5–1kg per week, which is a sustainable amount of weight loss.

Myth #5 – I will need to count calories

In order to have a healthy liver you do not need to count calories. This can be too stressful and time-consuming. You also want to avoid the detox to focus on the number of calories you have eaten rather than the quality of nutrition you are consuming. Most of us need to reduce our portions and this can be a visual process rather than a mathematical process as explained in the 7-Day Liver Detox Diet.

Myth #6 – It will be really hard because I will feel deprived

You should not feel deprived on the 7-Day Liver Detox Diet and it is not so difficult to follow that you feel like giving up. The goal with any lifestyle change is that it is sustainable. That is no different to the principles laid out in this book. Remember, however, that it can take

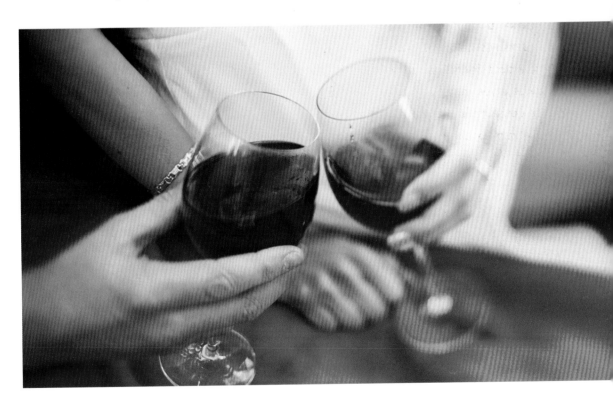

anywhere from seven to forty days for your body to acclimatise to the changes you are implementing, which can be a very challenging process for some people. Be rest assured, it does get easier with time, so don't give up!

Now that you are prepared and ready to continue with Your Liver Detox Plan the next step involves eliminating toxins that may be continuing to damage your liver. These toxins will continue to undermine your best liver detox efforts if they are not eliminated, so it is important that we look at strategies to reduce our toxin exposure before going any further.

Step Two - Eliminate Toxins

Harmful toxins are found everywhere (as fully outline in the chapter on 'Liver Haters') – in our diet, lifestyle and general environment. The build-up of toxins from all of these sources contributes to the toxic burden on our livers, leading to long-term damage. The key, then, when you are embarking on a liver detox program, is to eliminate as many toxins as possible to reduce this load. Below are some practical strategies to reduce the toxic load on the liver. They are broken down into the three main sources mentioned above: dietary, lifestyle and environmental.

Reduce Dietary Toxins

These include artificial preservatives, colours and flavours. These substances were not meant to be part of our diet and have been added to packaged foods to increase their shelf-life, palatability or appeal. Essentially preservatives are included in foods in order to sell more products, not to increase their nutritional value. The best way to avoid these dietary toxins is to minimise all processed and packaged foods, opting instead for fresh foods or homemade dishes. If homemade is not possible, especially because we are time poor, choose packaged foods that have been labelled as containing 'no artificial colours, flavours or preservatives'. Doing this will go a long way to reducing the burden on your liver.

Also avoid products containing mono-sodium glutamate (MSG), which is added as a flavor enhancer. This is sometimes labelled as flavor enhancer 621 on the ingredients list. This not only causes liver issues in susceptible individuals but also headaches, hyperactivity in children, a dry mouth, rashes, abdominal pains and irritability. Look for products labelled 'no added MSG', which will contain no or very little MSG. In the latter case the MSG found in the products will be the MSG found naturally in some foods in small amounts.

Other additives to avoid are artificial sweeteners e.g. aspartame, phenylalanine and sucralose. These are factory-made substances aimed at sweetening our foods without the calories that sugar contains. They promised to be the solution to not gaining weight but in fact have had the opposite effect. They are still thought to have an effect on the liver, as if they were pure sugar, and lead to fatty liver disease and weight gain. They are a toxin to the liver and are not natural at all. Avoid products containing artificial sweeteners and instead, if you wish to sweeten your food, try a small amount of honey, rice bran syrup or rice malt syrup. Keep in mind that these are still sugars and so use in moderation. Keep your intake to 1-2 teaspoons per day for the duration of the detox.

Sweet alternatives considered safe for the liver and not lead to weight gain are stevia and xylitol. Both can be found from health-food stores and most supermarkets. These can be added to baking and to tea and coffee. Keep in mind that they will still stimulate your taste buds like sugar and, in essence, keep you 'addicted' to sugar. If you are trying to reduce your sugar intake it is a good idea to slowly wean off all products that stimulate your taste buds towards sweet foods.

Other toxins found in food are hormones and chemicals such as antibiotics in animal products. Choose grass-fed beef and hormone-free, free-range chicken and eggs. Opt for organic where possible as these contain fewer chemicals than non-organic foods. As for fish, choose fresh and wild-caught where possible and opt for low-mercury containing species; avoiding those that contain a higher amount of mercury such as shark, orange roughy, swordfish and ling. Canned tuna also tends to contain high amounts of mercury due to the source of the fish as well as the size of the tuna caught (larger tuna species contain more mercury). If having canned tuna, limit to 2-3 small cans per week. Keep in mind that a healthy body and liver will clear mercury as long as it's not overloaded with mercury build-up.

Try not to store your food and drinks in plastic containers. Plastic containers can leach hormone-disrupting chemicals into the food, which can then enter our bloodstream. These have been linked to metabolic syndrome and infertility[18]. Where possible, store your food in stainless steel or glass containers. The same goes for water bottles. For lunchboxes, choose either stainless steel or BPA-free plastic containers. Avoid heating your food in plastic containers and avoid covering with cling wrap.

Reduce Lifestyle Toxins

Lifestyle toxins include substances such as alcohol and caffeine. The safe consumption of alcohol has already been touched on in the chapter 'Liver Lovers'. Alcohol excess is one of the major liver-damaging toxins. Keep alcohol to within safe limits. Drinking more than this will undo all your other diet and lifestyle efforts to stay healthy. Keep in mind that you may need to avoid alcohol altogether for a period of time if your liver is very damaged. Even if your normal alcohol intake is only a few drinks per week the liver may already be overloaded and unable to withstand further toxin insults.

As for caffeine, although it is a liver stimulant in small amounts and in a healthy liver isn't an issue, in an overloaded liver it can potentiate liver disease. The enzyme that breaks down caffeine in the body can work more slowly in certain individuals, even taking up to twelve hours to clear one cup of coffee or tea. Keep coffee as an occasional treat, to prevent liver issues just in case you are a person with the slow enzyme. You know you are this individual if you find it difficult to sleep after having even one cup of coffee or tea past midday. The speed of your liver enzymes to clear caffeine (as well as other toxins) can

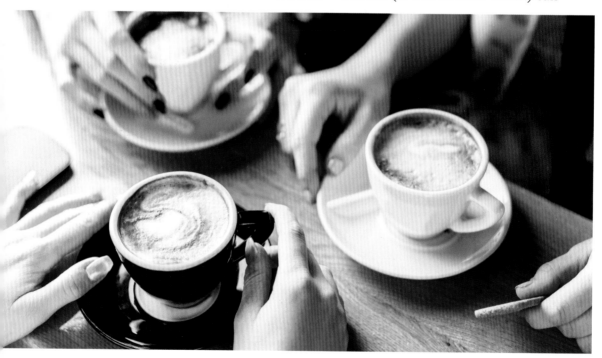

actually be tested via comprehensive liver detoxification testing. I occasionally undertake this testing but find that a comprehensive study of someone's dietary history will let me know how their liver is functioning.

The other lifestyle toxins that are commonly present are found in medications – prescribed and over-the-counter. Although many are safe, some can potentially harm the liver as mentioned in the list in the chapter on 'Liver Haters'. Minimise the amount of medication you are taking where possible. As your liver health improves you may find that you are able to reduce the amount of prescribed medications you are taking such as diabetes medication, cholesterol or blood pressure medications. This of course must be done under the supervision of your doctor but is a major incentive for many individuals to improve their liver health.

Reduce Environmental Toxins

Environmental toxins are those that we are commonly exposed to in our day-to-day lives and can overload the liver if cumulated. These include cleaning products, pesticides, cosmetics and personal-care products. Where possible, choose products that contain the least amount of chemicals possible. As for deodorant, choose labels that are aluminium-free. Aluminium is added to deodorant to prevent sweating under the arms but is thought to possibly accumulate in the body over time leading to health issues[19]. If you perspire noticeably, choose to only wear deodorant during the day and not apply it after your evening shower.

Choose organic produce were possible to reduce chemical load from pesticides in your fruit and vegetables. If cost is prohibitive go organic for lettuce, spinach, tomatoes, strawberries, blueberries etc. – foods that do not have a thick skin or peel that can be removed and, with it, most of the chemicals

Even taking your shoes off and leaving them at the door can prevent pesticides and other environmental chemicals from coming inside the house. Make your house and your body a 'chemical-free' zone as much as possible.

Now that you have eliminated a lot of the toxins your body and liver are exposed to on a daily basis you are ready to embark on your 7-Day Liver Detox Diet. Continue to follow the principles of toxin elimination to support your 7-Day Liver Detox Diet and liver health in general.

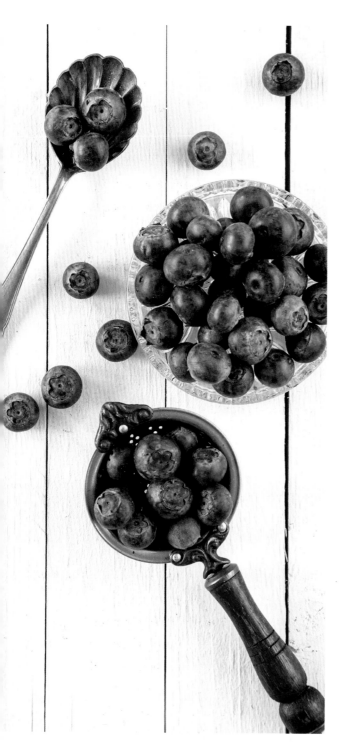

Step Three – Follow the 7-Day Liver Detox Diet

The following pages will now explain the 7-Day Liver Detox Diet, which is designed to detox your liver and optimise liver function so that you can have great liver health! This diet isn't a fad, nor is it meant to be a quick fix. It is, however, a tested approach in my clinic that gets results. It is not meant to be hard or time-consuming and has been designed with the busy person in mind.

All of the suggested recipes within the Detox Diet are able to be made within twenty to thirty minutes maximum. There are no unusual or hard-to-find ingredients in the recipes, but, rather, include commonplace healthy foods that we should all be eating anyway. To make it easier to follow, plan meals ahead of time and keep ingredients stocked up in the refrigerator and pantry so that they are at hand for a quick meal or snack. Although fresh ingredients are always best, if you need to freeze your meals so that they are available to take with you pre-made, then of course do so. Do whatever you need to do to ensure your success in following this plan! Your liver health depends on your commitment!

Why seven days?

This diet is meant to be easy to follow and so seven days for many of us is achievable to fit into and commit to in our busy schedules. It is also the minimum time required to see liver-health results. As previously explained in the chapter 'Know Your Liver' you may need to continue the 7-Day Liver Detox Diet for longer than one week depending on your Liver Health Score. If you have forgotten your Liver Health Score, take the time to now go back to that section and retake the Liver Health Questionnaire.

Although I don't necessarily enjoy using the word 'diet' it does explain that a level of change in eating patterns is required from your norm to shift your liver from sick to healthy. So here I use the word 'diet' loosely and would prefer to replace this with the word 'lifestyle' as, ideally, a whole new way of living could result from embarking on this Detox Diet and Your Liver Detox in general. Although it is normal to want to see quick results, it is a much better approach to think of change as a longer process leading to more permanent results. One thing is for sure – after the Detox Diet you will feel better.

So how will you feel?

As you follow the 7-Day Liver Detox Diet you may notice a few symptoms depending on your base liver health and current eating and lifestyle habits.

- *After 2 days:* Withdrawal headaches, breakouts, irritability, nausea, dizziness, difficulty sleeping

- *After 4 days:* Better bowel function, sweeter-smelling breath, less sugar cravings

- *After 7 days:* Brighter eyes, more energy, clearer skin, less bloating, better sleep

Do persevere through the withdrawal symptoms – that's just your liver detoxing and your body responding to removing addictive substances such as caffeine, alcohol and sugar. If you find that headaches are a real issue in the first few days, increase your intake of water and rest where possible. Try to avoid taking paracetamol and other painkillers for your headaches as this will undo all of your good work.

You shouldn't be overly hungry throughout the 7-Day Liver Detox Diet. Keep in mind that experiencing hunger between meals is actually a good sign. It means that our body is accessing stored fuel in the form of body and liver fat stores. Although it is encouraged to eat three meals a day with one to two smaller snacks to keep your metabolism firing, if you are finding yourself looking for additional snacks then consider asking yourself whether you are truly hungry or just bored. Take what has been coined the 'apple test' – if you are not hungry enough to eat an apple then you are not really hungry.

Keep in mind, too, that we often feel hungry when in fact we are just dehydrated and need a glass of water. Try in this instance having a large glass of water with fresh lime or lemon to see if the hunger abates.

If you are experiencing severe symptoms that last longer than a few days, speak to a healthcare practitioner. There may be an underlying condition that has been brought to the surface by the detox process that needs to be addressed, such as a metabolic disorder or diabetes. Alternatively you liver health may be so compromised and toxic and metabolic build-up in your bloodstream so significant that you may need extra liver support in the form of supplements or an altered liver detox approach that is beyond the scope of this book to discuss.

How do you monitor your progress?

As you go through the 7-Day Liver Detox Diet monitor your symptoms and become 'body aware'. As explained, you may initially experience detox and withdrawal symptoms but after a few days these should resolve as your liver health improves. Keep a diary of your symptoms before, during and after the diet so that you can review your progress. This can also help you stay motivated as you will see how bad you used to feel before undertaking the Detox Diet compared with during and afterwards. You may choose to use the 'Liver Symptom Tracker' in the Easy Reference Guide at the back of this book.

As for weight loss, many will notice a shift in their body weight within the first few days of undertaking the Detox Diet. This may initially be body fluid as the body starts to burn fuel stores and the liver and kidneys start to work efficiently. As your metabolism kicks in, body fat will be shed and with it liver fatty deposits, which will improve the function of the liver even further. This will then make it easier for you to lose more body fat as you continue the diet. Keep in mind that weight loss isn't always the best indicator of progress. It is definitely a side-benefit of undertaking the 7-Day Liver Detox Diet and having a healthy liver, but not the main benefit. The main benefit is how you will feel – healthier, more confident and less bloated and tired!

Sometimes the body is reluctant to shift body weight, especially if it has been holding on to this weight for a long time. Be persistent in following the 7-Day Liver Detox Diet and focus on these other benefits as your body continues to become more efficient at burning fuel. Eventually your body will release excess body fat stores when it feels healthy enough to do so. Don't expect rapid weight loss following the Detox Diet. Rapid weight loss is unsustainable and is mostly going to be body fluid and muscle loss rather than body fat stores. Do expect a loss of around 0.5-1.5kg weight per round of the Detox Diet.

If you are losing too much body weight during the diet then you may need to increase your protein intake. This may include an extra serve of chicken, fish, eggs, lentils or beans with breakfast, lunch and/or dinner. You may losing a lot of weight because you are undertaking a lot of intense exercise, which is not recommended whilst you are detoxing your liver, or you have a very fast metabolism. Try to keep exercise training to a moderate level while you are detoxing, that being no more than three times per week of high intensity training. Light exercise such as walking, gentle cycling and swimming, Pilates, and yoga is fine to continue to do regularly whilst you are doing the 7-Day Detox Plan.

So What is the Premise of the 7-Day Liver Detox Diet?

The 7-Day Liver Detox Diet aims to optimise liver health by following these principles of being:

- Low in fructose sugar
- Low in refined carbohydrates
- Low in bad fats
- Void of ugly fats
- Void of artificial preservatives, flavours and colours
- Low in foods that worsen iron overload
- Low in toxins
- Low in sodium
- Void of alcohol
- Void of caffeine and other liver stimulants
- High in fibre
- High in fresh produce
- High in healthy fats
- High in hydration
- High in variety
- High in Liver Loving Foods

The 7-Day Liver Detox Diet – Liver Friendly Foods

Here is a guide that complements your menu plan and can be used in addition to the list of good and bad foods as set out in 'Liver Haters' and 'Liver Lovers'. An explanation of how these foods will fit into your daily meals is provided in the section 'The 7-Day Liver Detox Diet – Day On a Plate'.

PROTEIN

Include 3 serves of protein per day with a serve of protein with each meal. A serve is a palm-sized portion of chicken, two palm-sized portions of fish or tofu/tempeh or one large egg. Keep protein lean and organic or grass-fed if possible. Do not deep fry, chargrill or barbeque your proteins. Lightly stir-fry or boil, roast or grill.

Include 2-3 serves of fish per week, including 1 of oily fish such as salmon or fresh tuna. Aim to consume 3-6 eggs per week.

BEANS & LEGUMES

Include 1-2 serves per day. Try replacing one serve of protein above for a serve of beans or legumes each day. A serve is a small handful or around 30g cooked beans of legumes.

STARCHES & GRAINS

Limit grains and starches to just 1-2 serves per day. A serve is ½ a cup of brown rice, buckwheat, millet, quinoa or amaranth or ¼ cup of oats. Gluten-free options such as bread and wraps are acceptable and preferable over wheat products if gluten intolerance is prevalent.

VEGETABLES

Eat as much veg as you like (minimum of 5 serves), but at least 1 serve per day of brassica veg such as broccoli, kale, cauliflower, Brussels sprouts and cabbage.
A serve is a cup of salad or ½ cup of cooked vegetables. Choose organic where possible. Choose fresh over frozen. Avoid microwaving. Steaming is best as this preserves the nutrient content. Vary the types of vegetables daily. Include a serve of fermented vegetables several times per week. With fermented vegetables, start with a small amount as they can contribute to bloating. If tolerated increase the quantity to ½ cup several times per week.

Vegetables can also be made into broths or soups but avoid adding any dairy or commercial stocks to your recipes. Avoid instant soups which contain very little nutrition. Also avoid canned soups as they often contain artificial preservatives, colours, flavours and MSG. If you need to add a stock to your recipe consider either making your own or choosing labels that are free of artificial preservatives, colours, flavours and MSG and are low in salt e.g. Massel low-salt vegetable stock (available from supermarkets).

FRUITS

Include fruit in the diet but limit to 1-2 serves per day due to fruits' high natural sugar (fructose) content. One serve is equivalent to one small piece or a handful of chopped fresh fruit. Some fruits have higher sugar content e.g. a medium-sized banana is equivalent to 1 1/2 serves of fruit. Opt for fruits that are lower in fructose, including berries, apple, pear, peach, nectarine, apricot or plum. Leave the skin on for added fibre, but wash well especially if the fruit is not organic.

Avoid fruit juice (even freshly squeezed juice) due to its high fructose content.

DAIRY

Limit to 1 serve of dairy per day as dairy may worsen fatty liver conditions, or choose dairy alternatives such as nut milks. One serve includes 200g of plain yoghurt or 200MLs of milk or milk alternatives. If you suffer from excessive bloating or wind, diarrhoea or loose bowel motions, nausea, heartburn or reflux, or recurrent ear, nose and throat infections consider choosing dairy alternatives instead of cow's milk products. Avoid soy milk and soy products as links have been made to an increased risk of thyroid health issues and certain cancers[20].

NUTS & SEEDS

Include 1 serve per day. A serve is one small handful or 30g of nuts or seeds. You can also choose nut butters but avoid commercial peanut butter due to its sugar and salt content. Try almond spread instead. Limit to 1-2 tablespoons per day.

OILS

1-2 serves of oil per day either as a dressing or in your cooking. A serve is 1 tablespoon of oil. Use cold-pressed and organic oils where possible. Avoid deep frying foods and instead stir-fry or grill.

HERBS & SPICES

Any unsweetened varieties of herbs and spices are allowed. Fresh is best but dried is also suitable.

DRESSINGS & CONDIMENTS

Avoid all commercially available dressings and sauces due to their additives. Do make your own as this doesn't take much time or effort and is much better for you.

SNACKS

Limit snacking to morning and/or afternoon tea. If there is more than a three-hour window between eating dinner and going to bed and you are hungry then also include a light supper from the list provided.

DRINKS

Drink 2-3L of water daily (filtered if possible). This should be your mainstay liquid during the detox program. You can choose unflavoured sparking mineral water. You may flavour your water with fresh lemon, orange, lime, ginger, mint etc. Limit juices to one glass per day of vegetable juice (with only a small amount of fruit added to make more palatable).

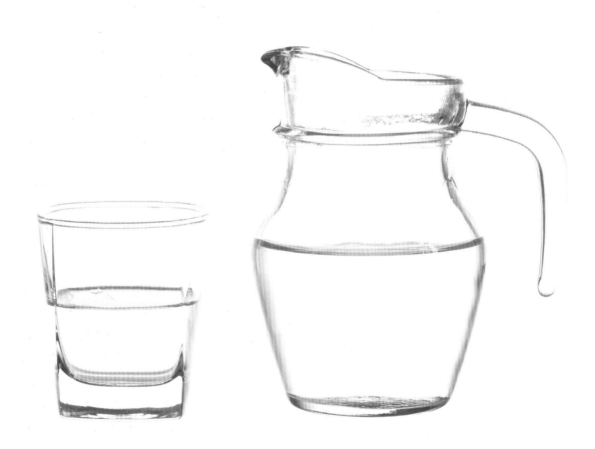

Alcohol, coffee and tea should be avoided. Once you have detoxed from these substances, which normally takes up to one week, depending on your baseline liver health these may be able to be added back in your diet in moderation. When re-introducing coffee back into your diet avoid café-style latte coffees as they contain a lot of milk. If you do buy from a café, choose the smallest size of coffee and order black coffee to which you can add your own milk. Do not add sugar to your tea or coffee. If you end up reintroducing alcohol into your diet keep it to safe limits to protect your liver.

The foods to be included in the 7-Day Liver Detox Diet are also listed in the 'Liver Friendly Shopping List' at the back of this book in the Easy Reference Guide. Take a photo of this list and carry it along with you when food shopping as part of your preparation to undertake your 7-Day Liver Detox Diet.

The 7-Day Detox Diet – Day On a Plate

On the next page are some further guidelines for breakfast, lunch, dinner and snacks to have during your 7-Day Detox. Of course you may choose your own options based on the guiding principles of what to include and what to avoid in the table provided.

Start your day with a large glass of water. Some find it easier to drink water first thing in the morning if it is at room temperature rather than chilled. Add fresh lemon or lime to taste. Wait 15 minutes if possible before having breakfast so that the water mixed with your food doesn't dilute your stomach acid and lead to indigestion.

Eat your meals sitting down and try taking 5 to 10 slow deep breaths before you start eating to switch on your 'relaxation and digestion' nervous system (parasympathetic system). This will aid digestion rather than lead to bloating and belching.

Make breakfast the largest meal of your day. Avoid skipping breakfast. Skipping this important meal sets the pattern for a day of overeating and grazing.

Lunch should be your second-largest meal of the day. If you find it difficult to eat a large breakfast, however, make lunch the largest meal of your day. Always include a large salad with lunch or dinner to ensure you are eating your vegetable quota for the day. Raw salad is also said to improve digestion due to the enzymes found in raw vegetables. If desired you may add 2 to 3 teaspoons of apple cider vinegar, which will aid digestion further.

Keep dinner as your smallest meal of the day. Try and have a gap of around 2 to 3 hours between eating dinner and going to sleep. Avoid carbohydrates with dinner.

Keep snacks for between meals when you feel hungry. Choose one to two snacks per day. If you find that you are hungry after dinner have a light snack of any of the following before bed. Avoid sugary snacks before bed as this will disrupt your sleep due to a peak and then a drop in blood sugar.

In addition to the snacks in the menu plan, you can choose from the following options:

- ✓ A small handful of nuts and 3-4 strawberries

- ✓ A small piece of fruit

- ✓ A small tub of unsweetened yoghurt with frozen berries on top

- ✓ Carrot, celery or capsicum sticks with homemade guacamole dip (lemon juice, avocado, pepper and sea salt)

- ✓ A handful of homemade kale chips, mountain-bread chips or unsalted corn chips with hummus (1-2 tbsp)

- ✓ 1-2 homemade protein balls (avoid using dates as a sweetener)

- ✓ 1-2 small homemade muffins (made with gluten-free flour alternatives)

- ✓ 1 corn or rice cake with 1 tbsp of almond butter or avocado

- ✓ A small handful of unsalted or lightly salted air-popped popcorn (pop in the frypan with no added oil)

- ✓ Freshly squeezed vegetable juice with any of the following: carrot, celery, cabbage, small green apple or orange, fresh beetroot, ginger, kale or spinach and/or fresh green herbs such as mint, lemon thyme, basil or parsley. Adding turmeric powder can assist with detoxification and inflammation. After juicing return some of the pulp to your drink for added fibre. Do add only one small piece of fruit to reduce the sugar content of the juice.

Drinks

Stick to water (still or sparkling) as your main drink. You may choose herbal tea or green tea (no more than 2 cups of green tea) throughout the day. Avoid drinking with your meal as this will dilute the stomach acid and interrupt digestion.

Drink before and after meals with at least a 15-minute gap between drinking and eating. Avoid drinking green tea after 3pm as the caffeine content may disrupt your sleep.

Portion control tips

If you are not feeling any better whilst following the 7-Day Liver Detox Diet perhaps your portion sizes are too big or have gradually crept up in size. Many people eat quite healthily but their portion sizes are very large. This will still overload the liver, even if the food choices on the plate are healthy. As a visual guide to what lunch and dinner should look like consider the following diagram.

Proportions of meal constituents on a plate

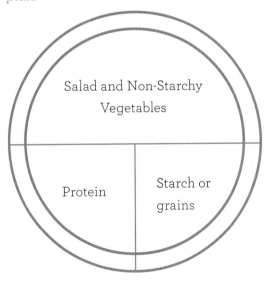

Consider that half your plate needs to include salad and/or non-starchy vegetables. One quarter of your plate can include protein and the other quarter starch or grains. You may include 1 tablespoon of oil or homemade dressing per plate of food.

Note that there are two rings on the plate shown on the left – an outer ring and an inner ring. A woman should aim for the inner ring on the plate which is around 2cm in from the sides of the plate. The outer ring is where a man or growing teenager would extend their meal. Keep plates small and consider eating off a bread and butter plate rather than a large dinner plate. The same goes for bowls – choose smaller bowls. Visually, the smaller the plate or bowl the more food it appears to contain, which may trick our stomach into feeling more full.

For more tips on portion control, including how to avoid mindless eating, refer to my first book, *Healthy Habits: 52 Ways to Better Health*.

Tips for eating out

When doing the 7-Day Liver Detox Diet you may find that it is unavoidable to attend certain social functions. You may also choose to eat out during the week for enjoyment. The problem is that food prepared outside of the home often contains more sugar, salt and fat than what you would normally use in your own cooking. The tips below will help you to make wise choices when eating out.

Choose	Avoid
✓ Fresh grilled fish without lemon butter or other sauces	✓ Heavy meats
✓ Grilled chicken	✓ Deep-fried, battered or crumbed options
✓ Garden or plain salads with dressing on the side or just olive oil and lemon juice as a dressing	✓ Heavy sauces
✓ Steamed or lightly stir-fried vegetables	✓ Caesar salads
✓ Vegetarian dishes such as dahl, bean stews and vegetarian stacks (without cheese)	✓ Curries
✓ Clear soups	✓ Pasta or noodle dishes
✓ Brown rice sushi with no added mayonnaise. Opt for tuna, roast chicken, tofu, vegetarian or salmon options (limit to 1-2 hand rolls or 4-6 sashimi pieces)	✓ Pizza
	✓ Creamy soups
	✓ Hot chips or potatoes
	✓ Alcohol
	✓ Breads
	✓ Burgers
✓ Sparking water	✓ Dessert or sweets

Special considerations (pregnant women, diabetics, children, elderly people and athletes)

Certain individuals should consult their doctor or nutritionist/dietitian before undertaking the 7-Day Liver Detox Diet. Pregnant women, children less than 12 years, insulin-dependent people, professional athletes and those who are frail due to age or chronic illness or disease fall into this category. If you are among these groups of individuals who have specific nutritional needs, I recommend that you see a professional dietician or holistic doctor, who may be able to offer some variations on the diet as well as guidance to make sure the 7-Day Liver Detox Diet will suit you.

Step Four – Choose Liver Supplements Wisely

The following table outlines supplements that may be of benefit in aiding and optimising liver health recovery depending on the level of liver damage (as indicated by your Liver Health Score – see chapter on 'Know Your Liver'). Don't overdo it with taking too many supplements. It is best not to overwhelm the liver and body further by ingesting copious amounts of tablets, powders and tonics. Stick with what you actually need.

In some cases it is best to consult your doctor to ensure that the supplements you are going to take will suit you and your health needs. Remember that everyone is different.

Liver Damage	Suggested Supplements
Mild	Silymarin (Milk Thistle) 1g daily
Moderate	Silymarin (Milk Thistle) 1g twice daily Vitamin C 1000mg twice daily Vitamin A 2500IU twice daily Vitamin E 400IU twice daily Vitamin B complex (containing vitamins thiamin (B_1), niacin (B_3), pyridoxine (B_6), B_{12}, and folic acid) Selenium 100mcg twice daily Zinc citrate or picolinate 25mg daily Magnesium oxide, citrate, or biglycinate 400mg daily Good quality fish or krill oil 1000mg twice daily
Severe	As above for moderate damage but add N-acetyl cysteine 500mg twice daily (as powder or capsule) as well as Co-Q10 (ubiquinol) 100mg daily and taurine 500mg daily.

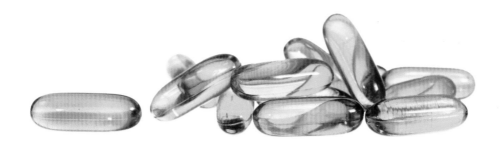

Step Five – Support Your Detox

In order to support your detox efforts and get the best results you will need to optimise the functioning of those organs that help to facilitate liver detoxification. As already mentioned in the chapter on 'Intro to Liver Health' the organs intrinsically linked to the liver and therefore very much impact on the function of the liver are the intestines, the kidneys and our skin. Suggestions on how to optimize the function of these organs are outlined below.

Intestines

A healthy bowel that digests and eliminates well will facilitate liver health. Digestion involves a complex system of internal mechanisms aided by enzymes and gut micro-organisms that help to process food so that all the nutrients are absorbed into the bloodstream and that the leftover products are then able to be eliminated from the body as faeces. Poor digestion disrupts this mechanism and can lead to nutrient deficiencies, which impacts our liver health.

Poor digestion can be the result of reduced enzyme and/or stomach acid production, from food intolerances or allergies, from parasites residing in our intestines, or from an imbalance of the good and bad bacteria that colonise our gut wall. These issues can lead to inflammation of our gut wall. As our liver is linked to our digestion by way of direct blood supply from our intestines to our liver, any gut-wall inflammation can release inflammatory toxins to the liver and potentially damage it. A sick intestine often means a sick liver. Do address these digestive issues, which often present as bloating, abdominal pain, excessive wind, constipation and/or diarrhoea, nausea and fatigue. Although not specifically addressed here, gut health can be improved by following the 7-Day Liver Detox Diet. If, however, you are still having issues, see your local doctor to rule out any more serious conditions.

A healthy bowel is also able to effectively eliminate waste. As touched on previously when we discussed gallbladder health, bile is eliminated via the intestines and so a healthy bowel will rid the body of this metabolic byproduct. That is, bile contains breakdown products of cells, hormones and cholesterol. If our bowel does not eliminate well then these waste products could be recycled and absorbed back into the bloodstream and back into the liver. This can cause both liver damage and other health effects such as raised bad cholesterol levels and raised hormone levels (namely oestrogen leading to weight gain).

To avoid this issue, it is important that we eliminate well and resolve constipation issues. Constipation can be caused by a sluggish bowel or one that spasms, or due to an abnormally long intestinal tract. Increasing our water and fibre intake can help resolve constipation as can taking probiotics and a small daily or second daily dose of oral magnesium salts (e.g. Epsom salts). Some of my patients swear by colonic hydration (colonics), whereby any hard or poorly eliminated material is flushed from the intestinal tract. The longer-term effectiveness and safety of this approach, however, is uncertain and I'm not convinced that it resolves the underlying issue. If you are still suffering constipation do seek help from either a nutritionist or dietitian or your local doctor.

Kidneys

In order to facilitate liver function our kidneys need to be efficiently filtering and removing toxins from our system. The kidneys are able to do their job effectively if we are well-hydrated. Drink at least 2-3L of water per day. This does not include water in tea and coffee or other caffeinated beverages but does include herbal teas that contain no caffeine. Observe the colour of your urine throughout the day to check how hydrated you are. It should be clear to light straw-coloured.

Skin

As toxins are also eliminated through the pores in our skin the easiest way to help boost detoxification is to sweat more[21]. Sweat pushes out the toxins to our skin surface along with water and salts. Exercise is an effective way to sweat as is having saunas. The best type of sauna for assisting with detoxification is an infrared sauna. These are very popular nowadays and can be found at many gyms and day spas. Make sure you rehydrate after you exercise or go in a sauna as you will have lost a lot of body fluid. The general rule is that for every hour of moderate-intensity exercise or for every thirty minutes in a sauna you need to drink an extra 1L of water. If you are finding that you are a heavy sweater and/or your legs cramp at night then you may need to add electrolytes such as potassium, sodium, and magnesium either into your water or taken as a tablet (found at chemists and health-food stores).

Some also advocate skin brushing whereby the dead surface layers of our skin are regularly removed by brushing the body. This is said to improve blood flow to the skin surface to improve detoxification but also to clear pores to allow for efficient sweating. Although the science behind this technique isn't confirmed you may find that using a dry or wet loafer on your skin during or just before a shower several times per week helpful in aiding your liver function. Many who currently practice this swear by it.

Finally, when looking to potentiate our best liver detox efforts we need to consider our thoughts.

Thoughts

Although not overtly linked with the liver, our mind can have a profound effect on our health in general, including our liver health. As mentioned previously in the chapter on 'Liver Lovers' one of the major contributors to liver disease in our society is having too much stress in our lives. Learning to deal with stress is one of the greatest gifts we can give to our bodies. Stress can lead to negative emotions. Negative emotions can have such a huge impact on our health long-term despite our outward efforts. Negative emotions can be a habit and, much like any habit, it can be broken with practice. Mindfulness meditation can be a great way to offset negative emotions by allowing us to become aware of our subconscious thoughts and thereby helping us to process our underlying frustrations and tensions. Taking time to reflect in this way can be healing as can taking the time to nurture our souls. Nurturing our souls can be achieved by any number of activities that we find truly restorative and enjoyable such as spending time with loved ones, walking along the beach, deep breathing, yoga, meditation, prayer, listening to music or just reading a good book in bed. Sometimes our negative emotions are rooted in bitterness, resentment, and an inability to forgive. In this case we may need to seek counselling support in order to learn to let go and move on and/or reconcile with those who have wronged us. Whatever the cause of our negative emotions, be they justified or habitual, we need to learn to manage them so that they don't erode our health.

With the above supportive strategies addressed and supplementing your 7-Day Liver Detox Diet you will well and truly be feeling your best! Your liver health by now will be at its peak and no doubt you will be reaping the health benefits. The next step in the process is to maintain your healthy liver so that your health can stay in tip-top shape.

Step Six – Maintain Your Healthy Liver

Liver health is maintained by following the principles outlined here and by following the premise of moderation as outlined in the chapter on 'Liver Lovers'. By following a Liver Loving Lifestyle your liver health can be maintained for life. This should ideally be your baseline lifestyle. Inevitably intermittent splurges will happen and that's when you may feel it necessary to follow the 7-Day Liver Detox Diet strictly for one week or several weeks to get your liver health back on track. But don't allow the splurges to go on uncorrected for months or even years at a time, as many seem to do. By allowing this to happen you create a build-up of toxins that will overload your liver again. You don't want that build-up to reach a point where the liver is so severely damaged that it takes many months of effort to return it to good health.

You may also choose to do the 7-Day Liver Detox Diet periodically throughout the year either to 'reset' your health or as a regular yearly goal. Let your symptoms guide you in whether it might be a good idea to do a round of the 7-Day Liver Detox Diet. Monitoring your health symptoms and being aware of what you are experiencing in your body is an important gauge of where your liver health may be. If you notice symptoms creeping back in that had disappeared whilst you were following Your Liver Detox Plan, then it might be a good time to get back on track and follow this section again. New liver symptoms may appear periodically, especially if you have let your health slip. In this case go back and undertake the Liver Health Questionnaire to see what your Liver Health Score is. This will inform you about the current severity of your liver damage and what you need to do to correct it.

Of course there is nothing wrong with doing the 7-Day Liver Detox Diet indefinitely as you may find that you feel so much better on it than off. This of course is ideal and if you can adjust your lifestyle to accommodate this new way of living then ultimately great liver and overall health is your reward for making a few sacrifices.

Inevitably, though, there will be those times when you splurge at a party or social function. The section 'Your Post-Party Detox' covers what to do when this happens and how you can get our liver health quickly back on track.

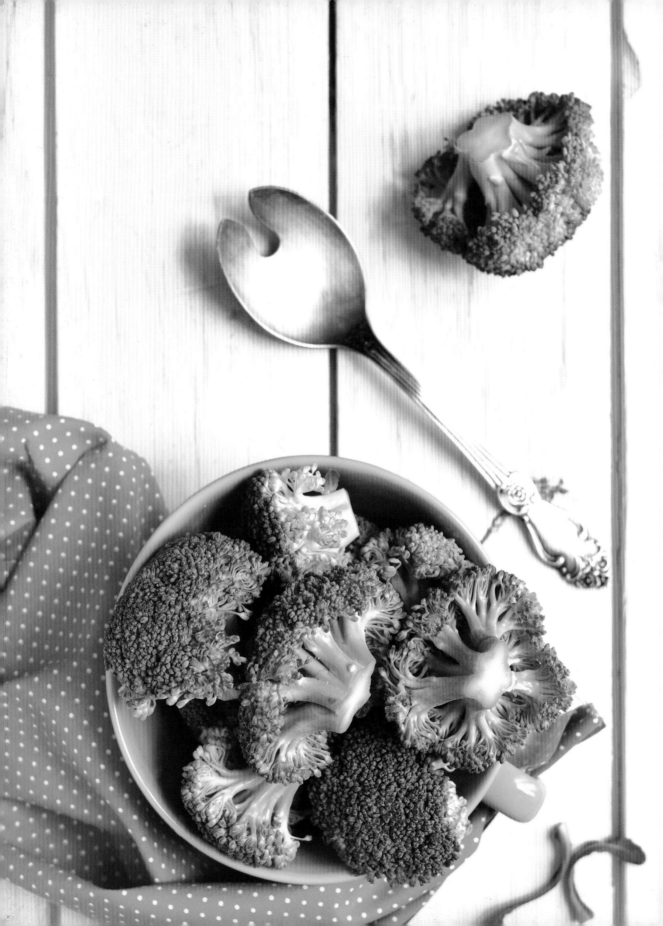

▶▶▶

7-DAY
DETOX
MEAL
GUIDE

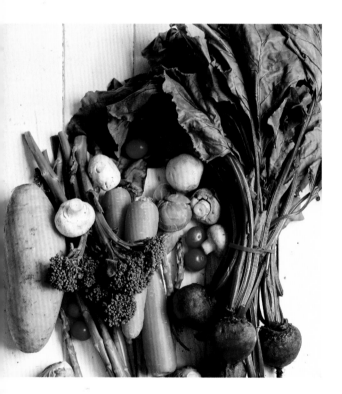

The following recipes are a guide to assist you with planning your menu for Your 7-Day Liver Detox Diet. There are flexible options for Breakfast, Lunch and Dinner as well as some recipes and a section full of tasty sweet treats. Smoothies are full of goodness and can be consumed at any time of the day. Our selection of salads can also be made to replace any of the Lunch or Dinner options. Feel free to add your own ingredients or change any of the suggestions here to suit your personal tastes. But make sure you follow the guide for healthy eating in the 'Liver Lovers' and 'Liver Haters' sections to ensure you are eating the right foods.

▶▶▶

BREAKFAST

▼▼▼▼▼▼▼▼▼▼▼▼▼▼▼▼▼▼▼▼▼▼▼▼▼▼▼▼▼▼
· ·

Breakfast is the most important meal of the day and will keep you going from morning till Lunch. Below are some delicious options for breakfast as well as some specific recipes:

Eggs

(Eggs are extremely filling and full of protein and omega-3)

Scrambled Eggs

With fried greens
Coconut oil, leeks, broccoli, spinach, mushrooms, chili flakes and salt and pepper

With avocado mash
Avocado, lemon juice, Himalayan salt and pepper, and cherry tomatoes

With fried mushrooms, tomatoes and zucchini

With goat cheese and mushrooms
Mix the eggs, goat cheese and mushrooms in a bowl and cook all together

Sweet Scrambled Eggs

2 eggs, 1 mashed banana, cinnamon, nutmeg and sea salt

Top with fruit of choice and a dash of maple syrup.

Breakfast Omelette

Tomato, mushroom and spinach with a side of avocado.

Asian style
Bean sprouts, carrot, mushrooms, chili, grated ginger and coriander. Topped with fresh coriander, fresh mint and lime juice.

Cereal

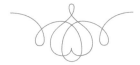

(Try any of these super healthy meals to kick-start your day)

Porridge

Prepare oats and add any of the following:

Grilled banana & cinnamon

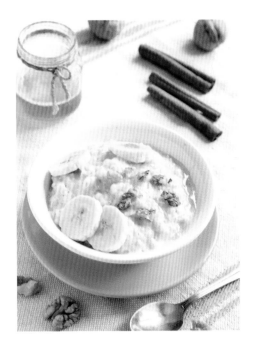

Grated apple and cinnamon

Chopped pear and raspberries

Strawberries and pistachios

Berries and shredded coconut

Natural peanut butter and honey

Recipes

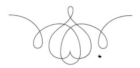

Bircher Muesli

Ingredients:

⅔ cup oats

1 cup almond milk (or milk of choice)

⅓ cup apple juice (no added sugar)

Dash of cinnamon

Dash of vanilla essence

Prepare the Bircher the night before by simply adding these ingredients to a bowl: oats, milk, apple juice, dash of cinnamon and a dash of vanilla essence

Leave, covered, in fridge overnight to enjoy the next morning

Top with fruit of choice and honey

Add coconut and top with cinnamon and honey

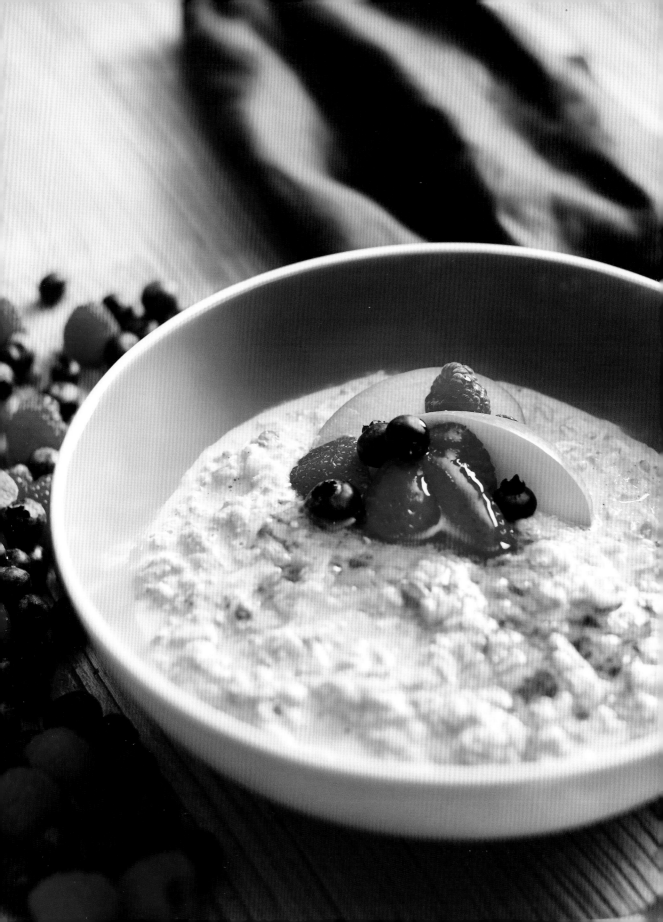

Protein Pancakes

Ingredients:

2 eggs

1 banana (mashed)

Dash of cinnamon

Coconut oil for cooking

Mix eggs with mashed banana and cinnamon

Heat coconut oil in pan over medium to high heat

Pour mixture into pan

Flip after approx. 4-5 mins or until bottom side is cooked

Cook on the other side and serve

Top with berry coulis:

Add some frozen berries to a pan over medium heat

Cook for approx. 5-10min or until the juices have thickened

OR add fresh strawberries and yogurt

OR grilled banana in coconut oil and cinnamon

Add 1 tsp coconut oil, sliced bananas and cinnamon to a pan over medium to high heat

Cook on each side until browned

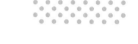

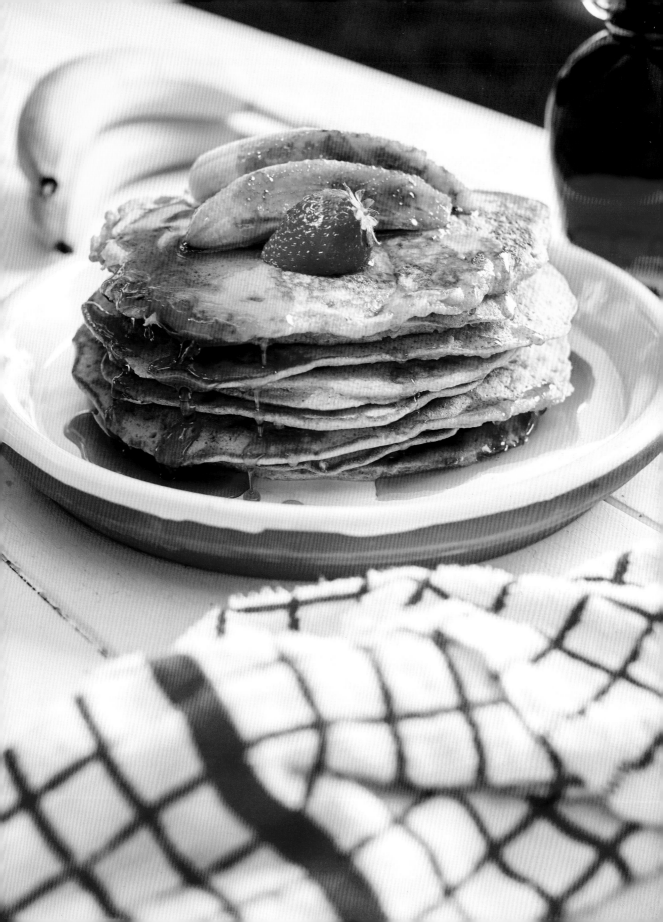

▶▶▶

LUNCH

▼▼▼▼▼▼▼▼▼▼▼▼▼▼▼▼▼▼▼▼▼▼▼▼▼▼▼▼▼▼▼▼
···

A hearty lunch will tide you over till dinner. Try any of these delicious suggestions:

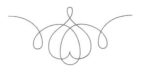

Chicken and Avocado Wrap

In a Mountain Bread wrap add:

Roasted or grilled chicken

Lettuce, tomato and cucumber

Avocado and hummus

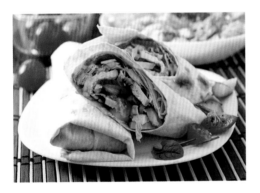

Scrambled Tofu

Pan fry tofu with cherry tomatoes, mushrooms, spinach, turmeric, paprika, cumin, cinnamon, salt and pepper

You can replace tofu with chicken

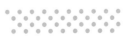

Recipes

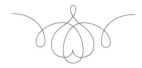

Roasted Root Frittata

3 roasted beetroots

1 steamed sweet potato

2 steamed carrots

10–12 eggs

Continental Parsley

Dill

Thyme

¼ cup Goat's Cheese

Salt and Pepper

Add vegetables to a bowl and add 10-12 eggs

Add continental parsley, dill, thyme, salt and pepper and mix

Pour into a lined rectangular tin and top with goat's cheese

Bake in a 170°C oven for approx. 20–30 min or until cooked through

Serve for multiple people or slice and freeze for a quick lunch on the run!

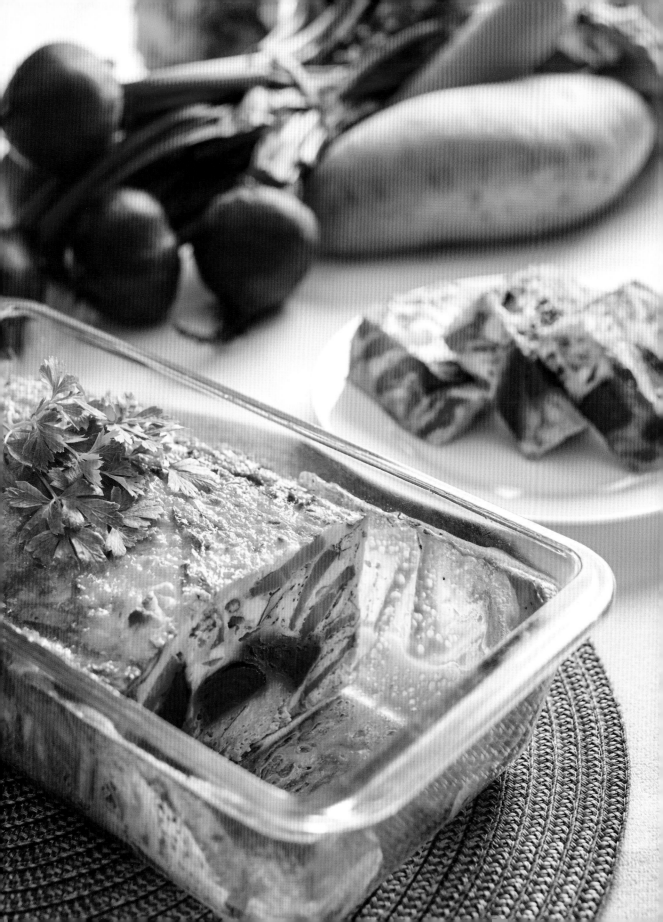

Veggie Patties

(These patties can be prepared in advance and frozen)

2 sweet potatoes (chopped)

½ cup grated carrot

½ cup grated beetroot

½ cup grated zucchini

½ cup finely chopped broccoli

A handful of chopped continental parsley and basil

Salt and pepper

1 egg

Preheat oven to 180°C

Heat a large pot of water over high heat and bring to the boil. Steam chopped sweet potato and cook until soft.

Add to a large bowl: steamed sweet potato, grated carrot, grated beetroot, ½ cup grated zucchini, finely chopped broccoli, continental parsley and basil, salt & pepper

Add egg and mix until combined

Roll combined mixture into approximately 15 palm-sized patties and flatten slightly

Fry or bake patties before serving

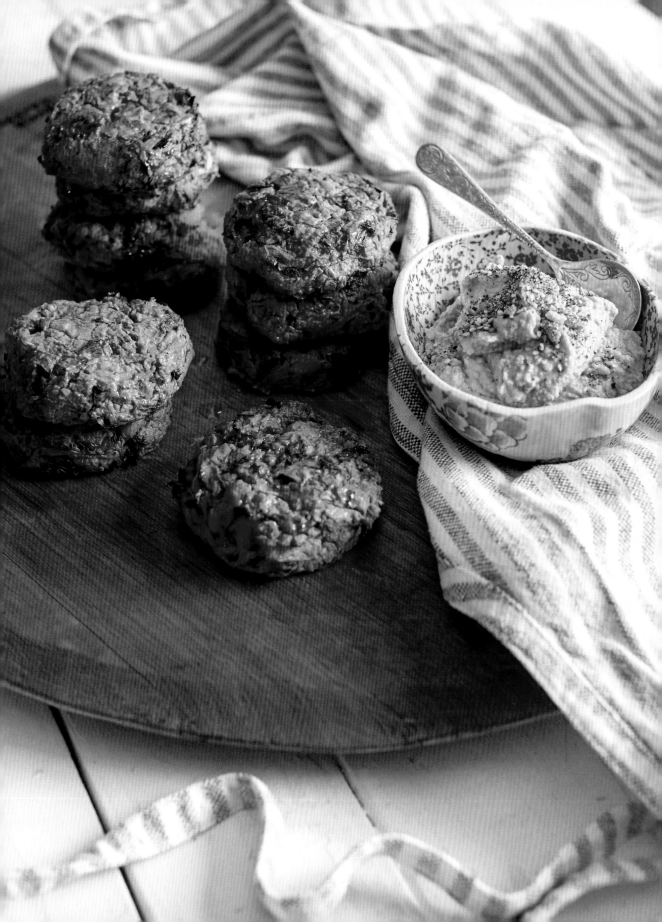

Pumpkin Soup

(Soups can be made in advance and either frozen or taken to work and heated)

4 cups chopped pumpkin

2 stock cubes (vegetable or chicken such as Massel low-salt vegetable stock)

2 garlic cloves

Pepper

Fresh coriander

Pepitas for serving

Bring a pot of water (approx. 1.5L) to the boil and add chopped pumpkin, stock cubes and chopped/minced garlic cloves. Cook until pumpkin is soft

Pour mixture into a blender

Add a dash of pepper and blend until smooth

Serve with coriander and/or pepitas and cracker pepper

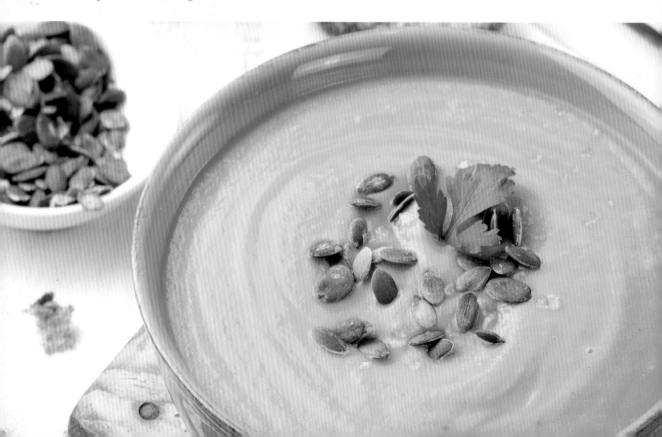

DINNER

Dinner needn't be a bland affair with these super healthy and super tasty meals.

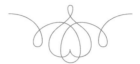

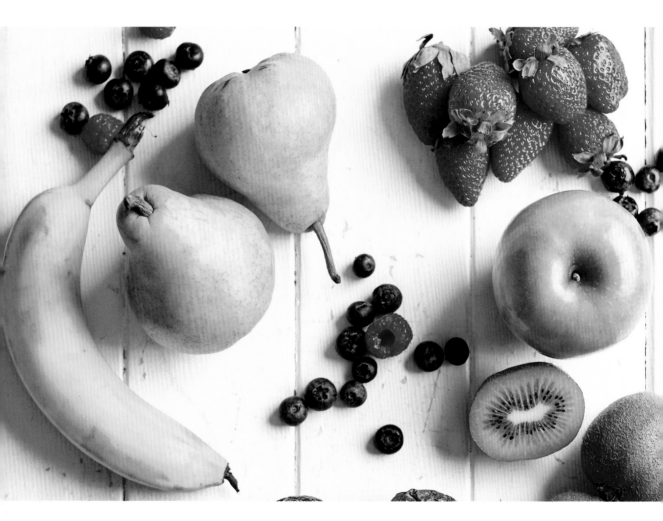

Chicken Stirfry

Carrot, capsicum and zucchini (sliced)

Chicken or tofu

Sauce: soy, honey and chili flakes
(2 tablespoons soy to 1 tablespoon
honey, and a dash of chili)

Serve with Brown rice or quinoa

Add cashews

Cauliflower Fried Rice

Cauliflower, peas, zucchini, corn and a
cooked egg (diced)

Add chicken

Add prawns

Stirfry with cooked rice

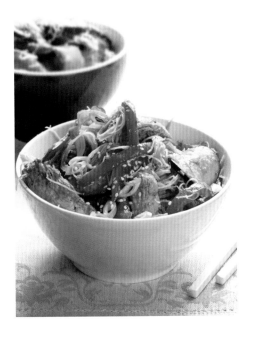

Recipes

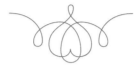

Chicken and Pineapple Curry

2 cups potatoes (chopped)

1 tbsp olive or coconut oil

500g chicken breast (chopped)

4 tbsp thai red curry paste

400g can coconut cream

½ cup chopped green beans

1 cup chopped fresh pineapple

Bring a pot of water to boil over high heat. Add chopped potatoes and cook until soft.

Heat a large pan over high heat and add olive or coconut oil and chopped chicken breast. Cook until browned and just cooked through.

Add curry paste, coconut cream, cooked potatoes, chopped green beans and chopped pineapple. Cook until heated through (approx. 15 min).

Serve with brown rice

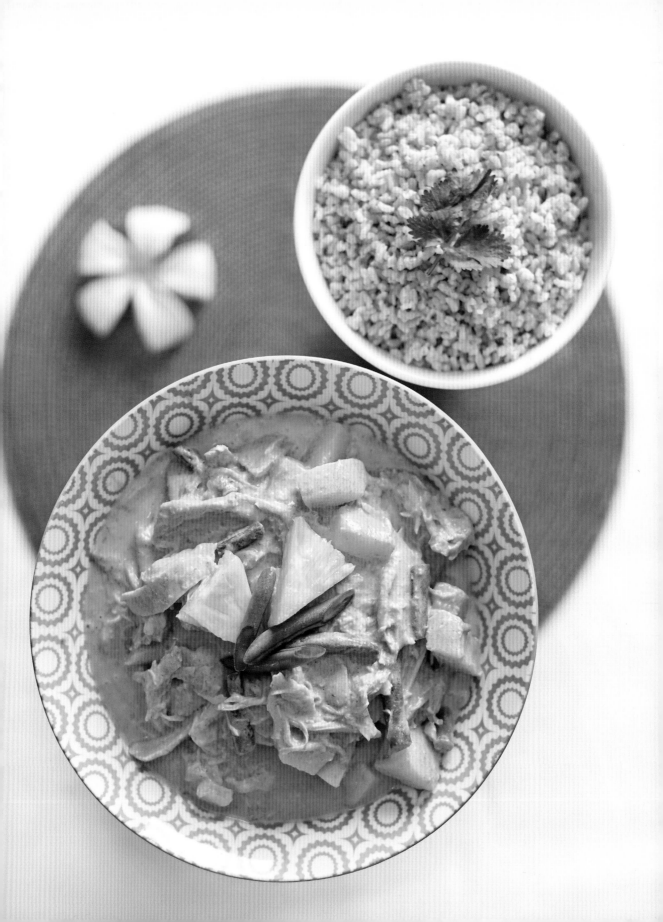

Almond Meal Crumbed Chicken With Sautéed Greens and Sweet Potato Chips

Ingredients

1 chicken breast (chopped)

1 cup almond meal

1 egg

1 leek (chopped)

2 cups spinach

1 broccoli chopped

½ tsp chili flakes

1 garlic clove (chopped)

4 tbsp coconut oil (or olive oil)

½ sweet potato (cut into strips)

1 tsp cinnamon

1 tsp paprika

salt and pepper

Preheat oven to 200°C

In a bowl add sweet potato, 2 tbsp oil, paprika and cinnamon.

Mix until sweet potato is coated and place onto lined baking tray. Bake in oven for approx. 20 mins or until golden and crispy.

In a bowl whisk the egg.

Coat your chicken pieces in the egg wash and then drop into a bowl filled with the almond meal to make a crumb.

Preheat 1 tbsp of oil in a large pan over medium to high heat. Add crumbed chicken pieces and cook on both sides until golden and cooked through. Season with salt and pepper.

Once you have removed chicken. Add 1 tbsp oil, garlic and chopped leeks. Sauté for a couple of minutes. Add spinach, broccoli and chili flakes. Sauté until browned and just cooked through.

Remove sweet potato from the oven and serve

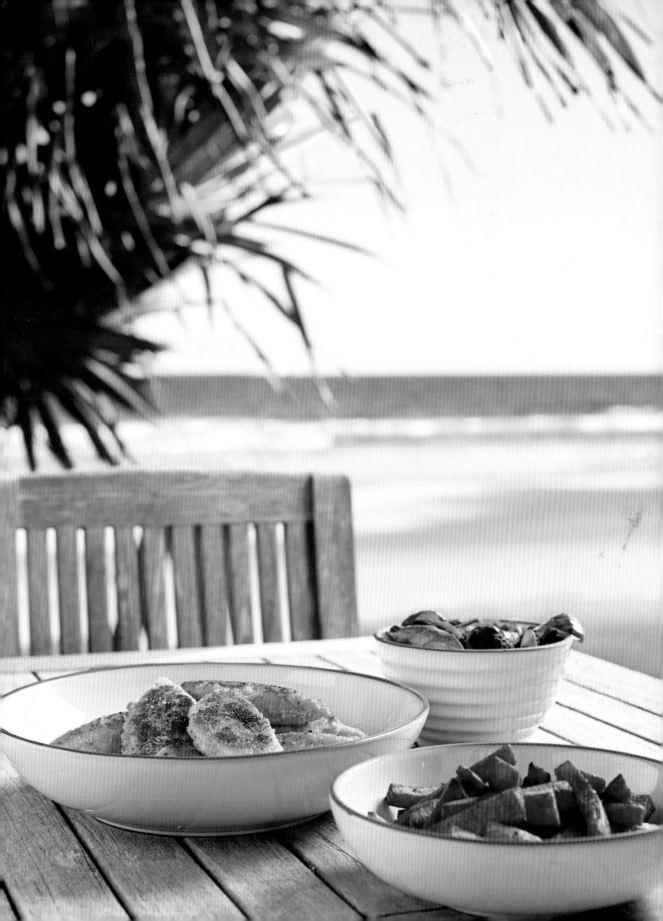

Shepherd's Pie

Ingredients

1 sweet potato

1 onion (chopped)

1 tbsp coconut oil (or olive oil)

200g beef mince

3 roma tomatoes (chopped) or 1 can chopped tomatoes – no salt

2 tbsp tomato paste

2 tbsp dried Italian herbs

1 carrot (chopped)

5 mushrooms (chopped)

Salt and pepper

Heat a large pot of water over high heat. Add chopped sweet potato and turn down heat to simmer.

Preheat oven to 180°C

Once sweet potato is soft, strain and mash with salt and pepper.

Preheat oil in a large pan over high heat. Add onion and sauté until browned.

Add mince and cook until just cooked through.

Mix through tomatoes, tomato paste, Italian herbs, carrots, mushrooms, salt and pepper.

Turn heat down to low and let simmer for 15min–45min

Pour Bolognese into a deep dish and spoon sweet potato mash on top

Place in oven for approx. 10 min or until the top is browned

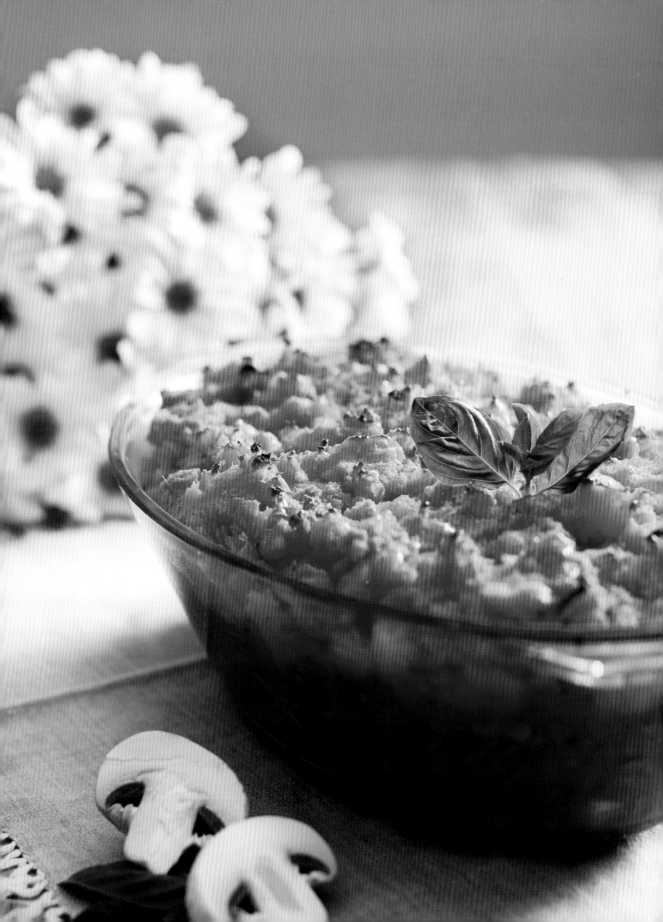

Chili Flaked Salmon with Roasted Cauliflower and Green Beans

Ingredients

200g piece of salmon

½ tsp chili flakes

1 cauliflower (chopped)

1 tbsp paprika

2 tbsp coconut or olive oil

salt and pepper

Handful of green beans

Goat's cheese

Handful of almonds

Lemon juice

Preheat oven to 180°C

In a large bowl add chopped cauliflower, paprika, oil and salt and pepper and mix until cauliflower is coated

Place on lined baking tray and bake for approx 20-30 mins or until golden

In a shallow dish add green beans and pour boiling water over and let sit for 5 mins

Drain and top with goat's cheese, almonds, lemon juice, salt and pepper

In a pan, over high heat, add salmon and cook on both sides for a couple of minutes

Using a fork, start to flake the salmon away. Keep turning the salmon and as it cooks, flake the outsides off the piece.

Once all salmon is flaked, add chili flakes, salt and pepper. Cook until crispy.

Remove cauliflower from the oven and serve with salmon and green beans

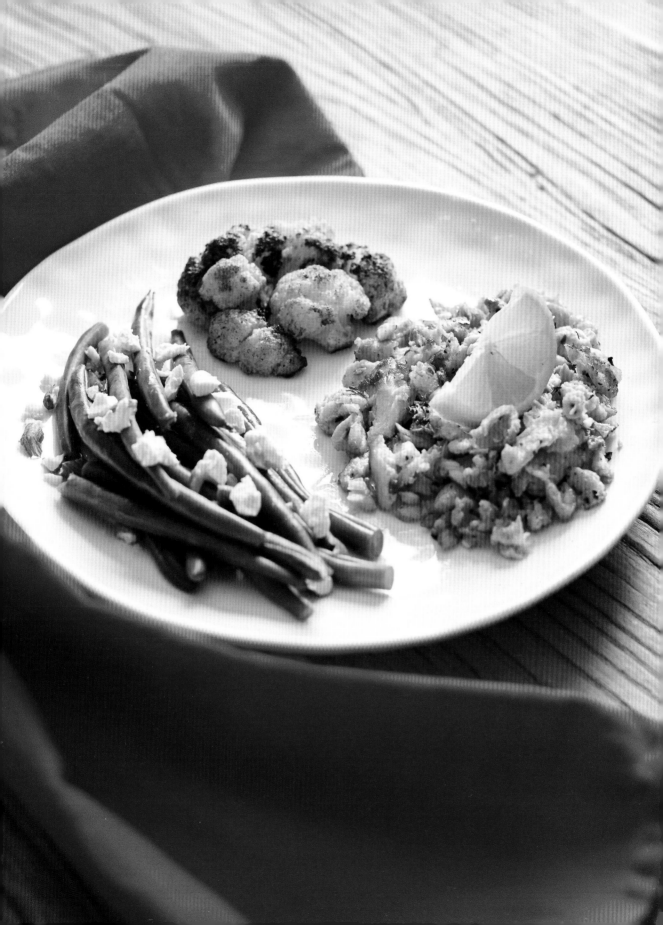

SNACKS AND DESSERTS

These treats are low in fat and virtually sugar-free. Keep some handy for when you need to ward off cravings.

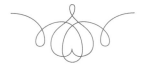

Protein Balls

Add 1 cup almond meal or blended oats, ½ cup almond butter, ½ cup coconut, ½ cup cacao and ½ cup maple syrup to a bowl and mix until combined.

Roll into balls and keep in the freezer for a quick snack anytime!

Hummus

Add 1 can of chickpeas, 2 tbsp tahini, juice of 1 lemon, 1 tsp cumin, ½ tsp paprika and 3 tbsp extra-virgin olive oil to a blender and blend until smooth. Add water if needed.

Beetroot flavour: add 1 roasted beetroot or 1 grated beetroot

Enjoy with chopped veggies

Guacamole

Avocado, juice of 1 lemon, salt and pepper. Mash with a fork and serve with chopped veggies

Chocolate Mousse

Add 1 avocado, ⅓ cup cacao, ½ cup coconut cream, 2 tbsp maple syrup and pinch of salt to a blender and blend until smooth.

Recipes

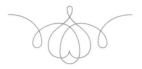

Banana Ice-Cream

Blend 1 frozen banana with ½ cup coconut water or milk of choice and ½ tsp vanilla essence until smooth

Add 2 tbsp cacao to make chocolate flavour

Add a sprinkling of crushed macadamias and shredded coconut

Top with berries or fruit of choice

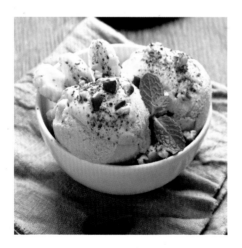

Homemade Chocolate

In a pot over low heat add ½ cup cacao, ½ tspn coconut oil and ⅓ cup maple syrup. Keep stirring until coconut oil has melted and mixed through.

On a lined baking tray, pour the mixture and add your choice of toppings listed below. Place in freezer for a few hours or until chocolate has hardened.

Remove from freezer, snap and enjoy!

Flavours
Pistachio and cranberries
Cranberries and coconut
Almonds chopped
Hazelnuts chopped
Frozen raspberries
Peanuts chopped
Fresh strawberries

►►►

SALADS

These salads can be made for Lunch or Dinner on any of the 7 days of Your Detox.

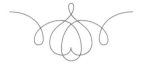

Asian Chicken Salad

shredded cabbage and carrot, radish, bean shoots, chili, coriander, mint.

Grilled chicken or roast chicken

Dressing
Lime juice, soy sauce and honey

Broccoli Tabouli

Quinoa or brown rice

finely chopped raw broccoli, cherry tomatoes, parsley and mint

Lemon, garlic and extra-virgin olive oil

Roast Balsamic Beetroot & Goat's Cheese Salad

Balsamic roasted beetroot

Broccoli

Goat's cheese

Roasted walnuts

Raw Summer Salad

Raw corn, greens, mango, avocado, cherry tomatoes, cucumber, mint and coriander

Lemon juice and olive oil

Salmon and Lentil Salad

Canned salmon, canned lentils, continental parsley, canned broad beans, rocket, sunflower seeds, olive oil and fresh basil

Roasted Cauliflower & Almond Salad

Roasted cauliflower with paprika & cinnamon, goat's cheese, almonds, spinach, Continental parsley, olive oil and lemon

Optional Additions:

Add grilled chicken

Add grilled/poached or canned salmon

Add canned tuna

Add 2 eggs

½ cup brown rice/quinoa/sweet potato

½ avocado

SMOOTHIES

Smoothies can be made any time of the day – for Breakfast, Lunch or Dinner – to replace any of the suggested meals. Or you could make yourself a smoothie for a tasty mid-morning or mid-afternoon snack.

Breakfast Smoothie

Nut Butter: water, banana, milk of choice, almond butter, sea salt, ice

Blueberry: water, banana, milk of choice, frozen blueberries (or fruit of choice), ice

Banana: water, banana, milk of choice, sea salt, cinnamon, nutmeg, ice

Mango: water, banana, milk of choice, frozen mango, ice

Mint and Lychee Crush

Add 1–2 cups coconut water or water, 4 lychees, small handful of mint and handful of ice to a blender and blend until combined.

Green Veg Juice

Add 1 apple, handful of spinach, ½ a cucumber, small handful of mint, ½ tsp grated ginger, juice of 1 lemon and handful of ice to a blender and blend until smooth

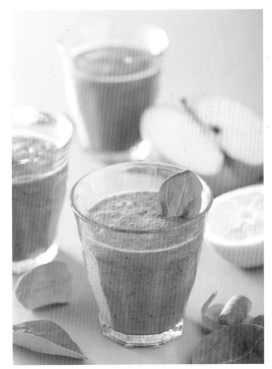

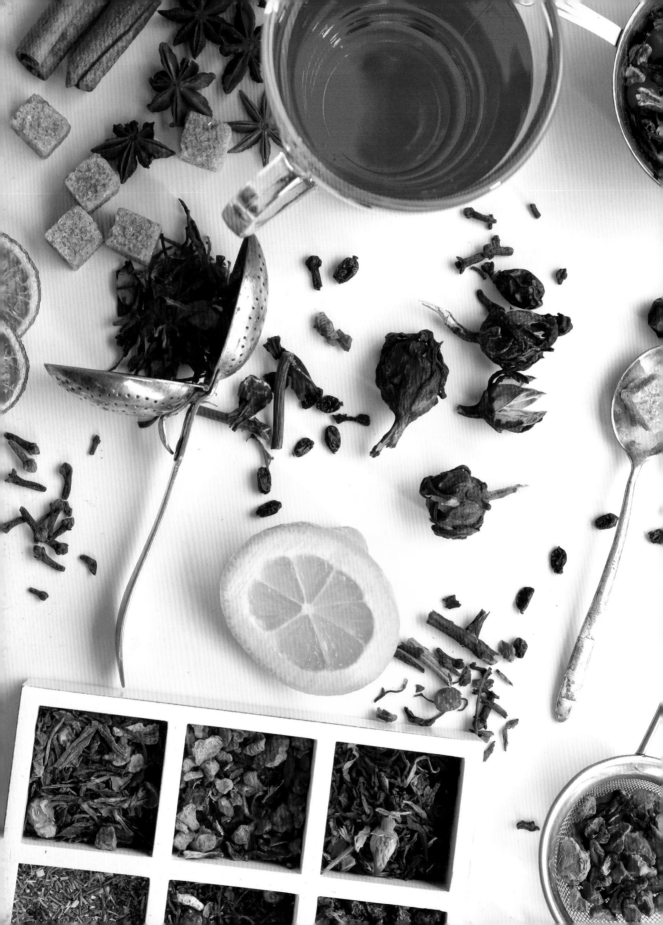

YOUR POST-PARTY DETOX

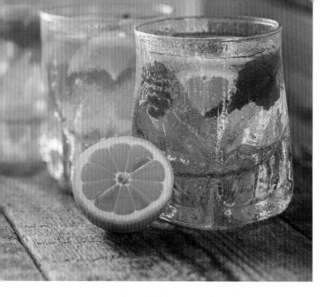

Party season seems to last all year these days with endless social functions and other commitments. There is a way to navigate these events so that your health doesn't suffer as a result of the overindulgence on food and drink. The key is to effectively 'detox' your system following one of these occasions so that these outings do not start to affect your health and waistline! Follow these simple tips for at least forty-eight hours following a party to help your body and liver recover and get back on track. These suggestions are ideal to follow if you have completed Your Liver Detox Plan and you are currently trying to maintain liver health.

Step One – Reduce Toxic Fats

The trans fats found in processed and packaged foods, as well as an excessive intake of saturated fats found in animal products (such as fatty cuts of meat), can overwhelm the liver's normal functioning. These can contribute to fatty liver disease as described previously.

If your liver is already overwhelmed by party food containing these fats, then for the next forty-eight hours avoid these processed and packaged foods (which is really a good habit for life anyway). Stick to good fats such as avocado, nuts and seeds, oily fish such as salmon and eggs. Avoid frying food in fats that can be converted to toxic fats as previously explained, choose instead macadamia oil, rice bran, grapeseed or a small amount of coconut oil.

Step Two – Hydrate Well

Provide your liver with the fluid it needs to eliminate and detoxify. Avoid further dehydrating you body by reducing tea and coffee intake to no more than 2-3 cups per day. Aim for 2-3L of filtered water per day for the next two days.

Step Three – Avoid Alcohol

This is especially important in the days following a big drinking session.

Step Four – Cut Back On Sugar

Fructose, found in table sugar as well as fruit, can overwhelm the liver if eaten in excess. The result, as explained previously, is fatty liver disease as well as insulin resistance. Since the body uses alcohol as a source of fuel in preference to other food sources while alcohol is still floating around in the system, it will store anything else you eat during this time as body fat. This effect can last for several days following a drinking session. So to reduce alcohol-related weight gain and the danger of contributing to fatty liver disease, keep your intake of sugar to a minimum following a drinking session. This means limiting processed foods, desserts and treats, which often contain large amounts of hidden sugars.

Step Five – Avoid Paracetamol

This medication is also processed by the liver. It is often taken for various conditions such as body aches and pains as well as headaches, including hangover headaches. If you have had a large drinking session and overindulged in party foods, my suggestion would be to avoid taking paracetamol for the next forty-eight hours following this as you may exacerbate liver overload. Stick to natural anti-inflammatories such as turmeric and boswellia.

Step Six – Stay Regular

A healthy liver requires a healthy digestive system as the two are intrinsically linked. Staying regular helps to aid the liver in its detoxification process and to help the bowel expel this waste. Keep your fibre intake high in the days following a party by including plenty of fresh fruits and vegetables, wholegrains, nuts and seeds. Adding psyllium husks to your breakfast may help to increase the fibre content of you meals without adding bulk.

Following the above tips will help to offset some of the effects of party overindulgence. The key of course is not overindulge too often! Still attend parties but keep in mind an important principle of good health, which is moderation. Note that a summary of these tips is also provided in the 'Easy Reference Guide' section of this book.

I realise that we all can cross our limit when we're in the spirit of partying and no more so than with alcohol. So how do we manage a hangover and avoid one in the first place?

Hangover Cures

Hangovers can be a nasty side-effect from drinking way too much alcohol and symptoms present differently for everyone depending on how much you drank, your age and gender, and even what type of alcohol you were drinking. Keep in mind that there is no such thing as a hangover 'cure' but you can avoid one in the first place and/or manage the symptoms if you find you have had a bit too much fun and overindulged. Let's first look at what actually causes a hangover.

So what causes a hangover?

The symptoms of a hangover from drinking more alcohol than your body can tolerate are caused by the following reasons:

- Dehydration – this results in headaches and is due to the fact that alcohol causes your kidneys to release more body fluids leading to large amounts of urine being excreted. This may also mean that electrolyte imbalances can occur and result in cramps.

- Stomach Irritation – alcohol irritates the stomach lining and intestine and causes inflammation. This can slow your stomach's ability to empty, leading to a sickly, full feeling. Increased gastric acid levels from alcohol consumption can cause nausea, heartburn and reflux. Long-term alcohol abuse can cause gastritis – a chronic inflammation of the stomach wall, which can lead to stomach ulcers[22].

- Toxin build-up – as alcohol is being broken down and detoxified by the liver a toxic compound called acetaldehyde can build up. This is thought to be up to thirty times more toxic than alcohol itself. This can cause liver damage as well as a fruity, smelly breath after a big drinking session.

- Brain Inflammation – alcohol may induce inflammatory markers called cytokines to skyrocket and these have been identified in body and brain inflammation and cause fatigue and memory issues[23].

How to avoid a hangover?

- Don't drink on an empty stomach. Before you go out, have a light meal. food will help slow down the body's absorption of alcohol.

- Don't drink dark-coloured drinks such as red wine if you've found that you're sensitive to them. They contain

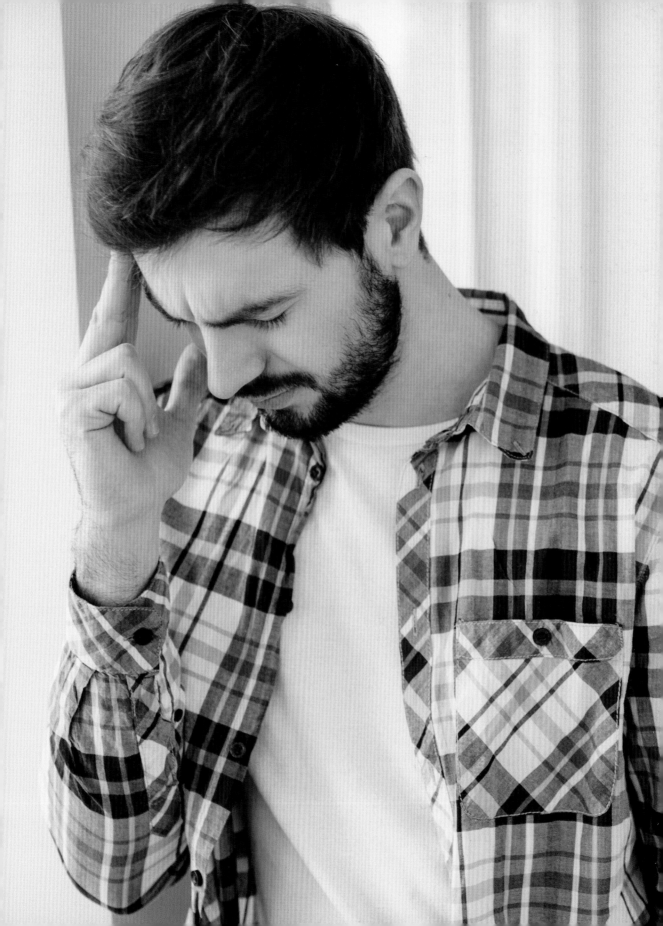

natural chemicals called 'congeners' (impurities), which irritate blood vessels and tissues in the brain and can make a hangover worse[24].

- Drink water in between each alcoholic drink. Keep in mind that carbonated (sparkling) drinks speed up the absorption of alcohol into your system.

- Drink plenty of water before you go to sleep. Keep a glass of water by the bed to sip if you wake up during the night.

How to Detox from a Hangover

Follow these simple tips to help you detox from a hangover. (Note that a summary of these tips is also provided in the 'Easy Reference Guide' section of this book.)

1. Start your morning with a large glass of water. Some find it easier to drink room-temperature or warm water with a little lemon added. Keep well-hydrated throughout the day by drinking at least 2-3L of water. If you experience cramping then add electrolytes to your drinking water – these can be purchased from chemists or health-food stores in powder form that dissolves. Some find vegetable juices can help with hangover symptoms. Avoid sugary drink and sweet juices as they contain sugars.

Freshly squeezed juices containing kale, beetroot, celery and ginger are a better option.

Aside from popular belief, drinking more alcohol does not help in easing hangover symptoms, it just 'numbs the pain'. Drinking in the morning ('Hair of the Dog') is a risky habit, and you may simply be delaying the appearance of symptoms until the alcohol wears off again.

2. Have a high-protein breakfast. Low blood sugar caused by a dip in alcohol levels can cause dizziness and feeling shaky. Protein helps to stabilise this dip. Your liver also needs the extra protein to heal and recover. Examples of a healthy, high-protein breakfast include eggs on a bed of spinach or kale, a protein shake or plain yoghurt and berries. Avoid processed cereals or fruit juices and avoid oily foods such as fried bacon, which can place an extra load on the liver and gallbladder.

3. Have a lighter lunch. Ideally just stick to a large salad with a small amount of lean protein. Include plenty of greens, which add nutrients without the extra calories and are also helpful in neutralising the acid produced by the alcohol in the body.

If you find that you just can't stomach having a solid lunch then try bouillon soup. A thin vegetable-based broth is also a good source of vitamins and minerals, which can top up depleted resources. The main advantage of a simple soup is that it's easy for a fragile stomach to digest. This dish can be homemade or purchased from supermarkets or health-food stores as cubes that dissolve in water.

4. Trade coffee for herbal tea. Coffee can place a strain on the liver's ability to detoxify and, although it may make you feel better initially, can actually make you feel worse as the day goes on. Since alcohol can disrupt the quality of your sleep, avoiding coffee for at least twenty-four hours following a hangover can assist you in getting a good night's sleep the day after.

5. Make your evening meal the smallest of the day. Opt for fresh steamed vegetables and fish or chicken. Avoid fatty cuts of meat and heavy sauces. Eat your dinner at least two hours before bed to allow proper digestion.

6. Avoid dessert. Have a herbal tea instead and avoid having any more alcohol. Trade the glass of wine for sparkling mineral water.

By following these tips, party season can be less damaging to our health and help us to enjoy ourselves to the full without the long-term consequences to our liver and waistlines!

The following chapter explores some interesting liver case histories from my clinical practice that you or someone you know may be able to relate to. These stories may help to consolidate the information you have learnt in this book and guide you on your own liver health recovery.

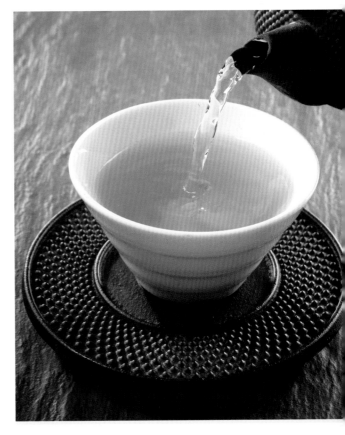

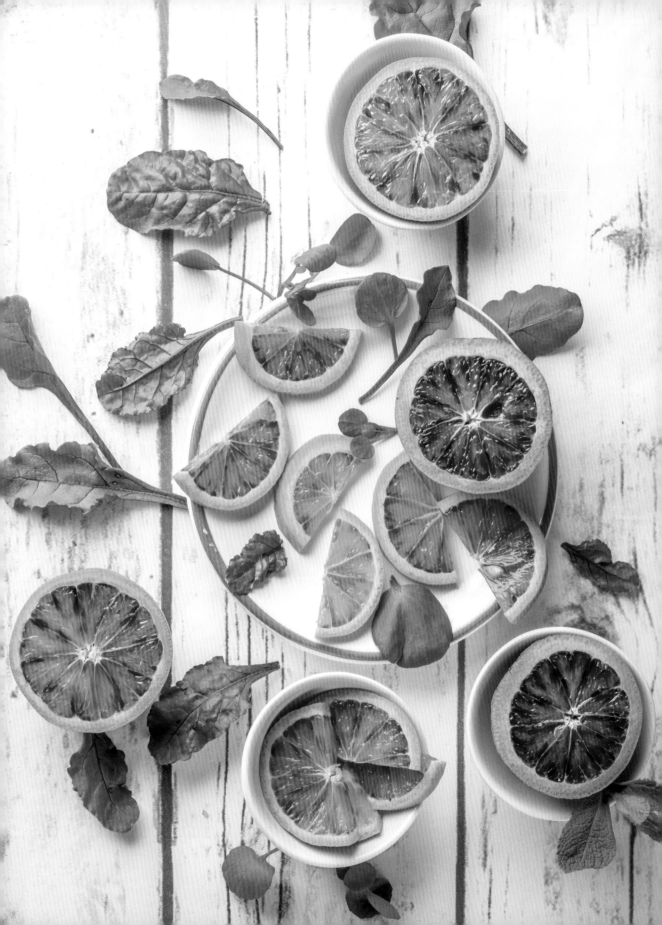

INTERESTING LIVER CASES

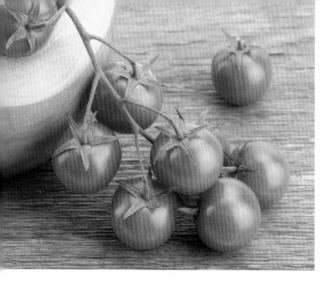

To make it easier to relate to the information provided in this book I have outlined several interesting cases that reveal common problems that I see in clinical practice. These cases are based on actual patients with liver conditions, but their names and any specific information that identifies them has been changed to protect their privacy. These patients are just like you and me – real people living in today's busy world, trying to do their best but not realising that their health is suffering as a consequence of some of the decisions they are making on a regular basis. It is easy to see how our liver health in particular can suffer from these decisions, especially when we examine them from a birds-eye perspective.

Keep in mind that not every case history may relate to you but at least one is likely to resonate. Studying these case histories may offer insight into how you

may recover your health. By following the simple strategies in this book, the patients below were able to turn their liver health and overall wellbeing around for the better. Use their stories as motivation that you too can improve your wellbeing and live a healthier life.

Liver Case # 1 – The Hormone Storm

Helen is a 57-year-old woman who had always had relatively good health. That is until menopause, when symptoms really hit her hard. She suffered from hot flushes and sweating profusely during the day but particularly at night, which was interfering with her quality of sleep. She felt tired a lot of the time and irritable. Her husband had noticed a change in her personality and had mentioned that she wasn't as patient and happy as she used to be. Her libido had dropped significantly and this was also causing problems in her relationship. One thing that bothered Helen greatly was that she previously had never had a problem with her weight but since going through menopause she had gained about six kilograms and noticed that it was mainly around her mid-section. She no longer felt attractive or healthy even though her exercise regimen had not changed. She put up with her symptoms for about eighteen months until she decided that she had to do something.

She saw her local GP who prescribed hormone-replacement therapy after discussing the risks with her. She decided that her quality of life was worth the risk and so she started on this treatment right away. Within a few days her hot flushes had resolved and her mood had improved slightly, which she attributed to finally getting a full night's sleep, but she still did not lose any weight. In fact, she felt like she was gaining even more weight. Other symptoms started to appear and she noticed that her feet had begun to swell, especially in the evenings. She suffered mild nausea most days and noticed that she also suffered frequent headaches. Most days she just didn't feel well and wondered if there was something really wrong with her. Over the next few years she felt like she had aged very quickly.

That's when she presented to me wondering if there was something that she could do to feel well again. I examined Helen and noticed that she had slightly reddened palms, dark circles under her eyes, and a thick coating on her tongue, which I was able to scrape off with a spatula. Her abdomen was generally bloated and slightly tender under her right ribs. Her feet were puffy but not overly swollen with fluid. Her blood pressure was 130/85, which is slightly elevated. I queried Helen's symptom history and undertook a Liver Health Questionnaire with her. She scored 20, which just saw her in the 'Moderate Liver Damage' category. The largest individual question score for Helen was the alcohol consumption question, where she scored a 3. In the last few years she had been drinking at least 3 glasses of wine at night to unwind from her day and to deal with family stress.

I asked Helen to have some blood tests and a liver ultrasound due to the tenderness she felt when I had examined her. Her liver function results are shown below (the normal laboratory references ranges are shown in brackets):

- Total bilirubin 18 (2-24) – normal result

- ALP 67 (30-110) – normal result

- GGT 76 (<60) – slightly elevated

- ALT 65 (<55) – slightly elevated

- AST 55 (<45) – slightly elevated

Helen's liver ultrasound indicated that she had fatty liver disease with no gallbladder disease or gallstones. All other testing was within normal ranges.

I explained the results to Helen and told her that I felt that her symptoms were largely caused by liver damage. I felt that her liver was being overloaded by some of her lifestyle choices, including too much alcohol. I also felt that the hormone-replacement therapy was potentially also having an impact on her liver as can be the case with oral forms (tablets or capsules) of hormone therapy.

The synthetic forms of progesterone in hormone therapy (as well as the oral contraceptive pill) can also overload the liver.

I suggested we switch her over to a hormone cream for her hormone replacement therapy as this does not have to be processed by the liver. I also suggested that she trial the 7-Day Liver Detox Diet along with cutting out alcohol for one month. I also prescribed a liver support supplement (St Mary's Thistle). After only seven days she felt a lot better. She had a lot more energy, her eyes were clearer, and she was sleeping more soundly than before. She felt so good that she decided to follow the 7-Day Liver Detox Diet for an entire month.

Following this, Helen had a blood test to review her results. Her liver markers were:

- Total bilirubin 18 (normal)

- ALP 67 (normal)

- GGT 55 (normal)

- ALT 45 (normal)

- AST 42 (normal)

She was ecstatic that her results indicated that her liver health was returning to normal. I explained that her results were still at the higher end of normal and that she should continue her new, healthier habits for another month. She did so willingly as she found that she felt so much better. After two months of following the above suggestions Helen's results were completely back within the healthy normal range. A repeat liver ultrasound showed that the fatty liver was clearing and her liver was no longer completely infiltrated by fatty streaks. Helen had also lost 3kg and her libido had also improved. Her blood pressure had returned to a healthy range of 118/75. She no longer felt overloaded and 'toxic' as she called it. Helen continues to follow these suggestions and now has the occasional glass of wine on the weekends but has fortunately not slipped back into old habits.

Liver Case #2 – Too Tired for Too Long

Rachel is a 34-year-old mother of two who had been feeling very run down for the previous two years but particularly in the previous three months. She came to see me hoping that I would be able to find out why she was feeling so bad. Although she hadn't had any blood tests for a while, Rachel's previous tests at her local GP had always come back normal. Her fatigue was so severe that she often felt like going to bed within two hours of waking up in the mornings.

I asked Rachel if any other symptoms had appeared around the time of the fatigue. Rachel mentioned that she had been feeling quite anxious and although she was quite tired at the end of the day she was unable to switch off her thoughts and fall asleep at night. She tossed and turned all night and then finally fell asleep in the early hours of the morning only to be woken by her young children. She often felt hot and itchy at night and had gained around 10kg in the last two years. She felt bloated and alternated between being constipated and having loose bowel motions. She was using chocolate to get through the day and it wasn't unusual for Rachel to eat a small family block of chocolate a day.

Rachel didn't have any energy to exercise, and even if she did she explained that she simply didn't have the time. Her husband was working away and was home one week out of the month and so she was responsible for looking after the kids and home as well as working part-time. She mentioned that they had been under a lot of financial stress in the last two to three years and her husband had to take an interstate job to cover the bills. She lacked social support, often felt very frustrated at the lack of personal time, and was often lonely. She felt she needed to change some habits but did not know where to start. We undertook the Liver Health Questionnaire and Rachel's Liver Health Score came to 18 indicating possible mild liver damage.

I examined Rachel and found that she had a low blood pressure of 95/66. This was causing her to feel dizzy and lightheaded on occasions, especially when she stood up. She looked very pale and had some other physical signs of anaemia. Her abdomen was tender everywhere. She had some bruises to her legs and forearms but could not remember how these happened. She said that she bruised easily. Her tongue was coated and there were cracks at the sides of her lips. Rachel mentioned she was often prone to cold sores. Her feet, ankles and legs were generally very puffy. She had bumps on the backs of her arms like tiny pimples (sign of zinc deficiency and/ or gluten intolerance). Rachel said they had been there for at least six months. Overall, Rachel's health was really suffering and she had general signs of liver overload and malnourishment. Her body was simply not able to utilise the nutrients in her food because of her poor digestion and liver health.

I explained to Rachel what I felt was going on with her health and how I thought that stress may have initially triggered her symptoms. I mentioned to her that she needed to have some testing to rule out any serious conditions before I offered my suggestions on how to help her get her health back on track. Rachel agreed and had some blood tests, a urine test for iodine levels, as well as a salivary hormone test.

The blood tests revealed that she was slightly low in iron stores leading to mild iron-deficiency anaemia, had slightly low vitamin B12 levels, and was low in vitamin D, zinc and iodine. These are all common deficiencies of someone who has been under stress for a long time. Her thyroid function was normal, ruling out a thyroid condition as was any other markers of autoimmune diseases. Her liver function testing revealed the following:

- Total bilirubin 18 (normal)

- ALP 67 (normal)

- GGT 35 (normal)

- ALT 56 (slightly elevated)

- AST 62 (slightly elevated)

This indicated that Rachel's liver was overloaded and potentially heading toward fatty liver disease. The overload in Rachel's case was from stress, poor digestive health, as well as the extra weight that she was carrying.

Rachel's salivary hormone testing revealed that she had very low cortisol reserves, a sign of chronic stress, and explained why she felt so exhausted. Her oestrogen levels were elevated, which caused her to retain fluid, and her progesterone levels were relatively low, causing her to feel anxious.

I explained all of these results to Rachel and suggested that she following the 7-Day Liver Detox Diet for at least two weeks. Although she was not coeliac on her blood testing I thought that perhaps she was gluten-intolerant given her symptoms and asked her to follow the diet but choose gluten-free options. I also suggested some supplements to correct her deficiencies and asked that she find time to rest as much as possible, leaving the housework on occasion. I also prescribed a supplement to help her liver process the extra oestrogen from her system (brassica extract) as well as a liver support supplement (St Mary's Thistle).

I did not see Rachel for two months and almost didn't recognise her when she

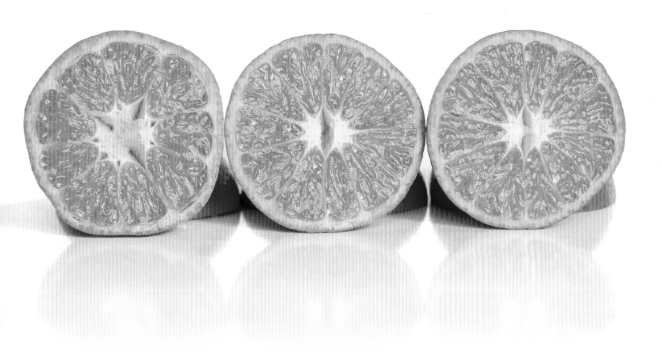

did present back at the clinic. She said that she had planned to return sooner but had been busy with the kids. She had continued to follow my suggestions for the entire time. She was much happier and seemed to be carrying a lot less fluid. She was no longer puffy in the legs or face. Her eyes were brighter and the dark circles under her eyes had gone. She mentioned that she had much less trouble with her bowels. She had lost around 2-3kg and felt a lot less bloated. She was a lot more confident and stated that she now had energy to get through her day as well as to exercise two days per week. Her whole lifestyle had changed and she was no longer relying on chocolate to get by. Her repeat blood results reflected her improvement. All her vitamin and mineral deficiencies had resolved and her liver markers had returned to normal.

The last time I saw Rachel, which was nine months after her initial consultation, she had completely changed her lifestyle because it made her feel so much better. She had reduced her stress levels where possible and was still following the Detox Plan but was allowing herself to have the occasional splurge on the weekends at parties or family gatherings. She was a much happier, healthier version of herself.

Liver Case #3 – An Aussie Issue

Bill is a 63-year-old man who was nearing retirement when he came to see me, but was not feeling well enough to enjoy his last few years of working life. He had been under a lot of pressure with his business and felt the need to continue to work long hours to sustain his profitability so that he could sell the business and retire comfortably. He had had poor health for the last five years and had been to see several specialists, who all warned Bill that he needed to make some drastic changes to his lifestyle. For much of his life Bill had used alcohol to relax as well as to socialise. He had been drinking consistently since he was 17 years old and particularly heavily in the last five years. It was not unusual for Bill to finish a bottle of wine each night as well as two to three beers and a 'Johnnie Walker' before bed to help him sleep.

He had suffered from depression since his divorce ten years previously and was on two different forms of anti-depressant medication. He often felt overwhelmed and frustrated. He had gained 20kg in the last ten years and had been diagnosed with metabolic syndrome recently by another doctor. He knew that his drinking was an issue but he just wasn't sure how he could change his behaviour since he had been drinking for so long. I explained to Bill that his case was not unusual. Many Australian men have the same issue. I believed he could turn his health around with some help.

On examination Bill was very overweight with most of the extra weight sitting around his mid-section. He was grey in appearance and had dark circles under his eyes. He had broken capillaries across his nose and cheeks that gave them a flushed appearance. Broken capillaries often appear in the faces of those who drink heavily. He spoke softly and often looked down as if ashamed by his appearance. His blood pressure was 145/90, which put him at higher risk of heart disease and stroke. His abdomen was generally tender especially under his right ribs in the region of his liver. He did not have any ankle swelling but did have red marks across his chest that he mentioned had only been there for the last two years. These had the appearance of liver spots or telangiectasia.

I asked Bill to have some blood tests as well as a liver ultrasound. His results indicated that he had markedly elevated liver enzymes:

- Total bilirubin 25 (slightly elevated)

- ALP 150 (elevated)

- GGT 320 (elevated)

- ALT 250 (elevated)

- AST 190 (elevated)

His urea levels were also elevated indicating an increased risk of gout. His blood sugar levels and bad cholesterol levels were also elevated putting him at increased risk of heart disease. He had slight vitamin B12 deficiency. He had slightly delayed clotting as indicated on coagulation testing – a sign of more severe liver damage. He had low albumin stores (a body transport protein the liver makes) – also a sign of severe liver damage. His iron stores were extremely elevated at 1200, which made me think that he may have hereditary haemachromatosis. This was subsequently ruled out on genetic testing and so the elevated iron stores were put down to liver damage. His liver ultrasound indicated a diffusely damaged liver that had started to shrink due to the damage.

I explained the results to Bill and mentioned that he needed to change his lifestyle asap to avoid a heart attack and further damage to his health. I explained that I thought his liver was severely damaged and that I suspected he might already have cirrhosis of the liver. To diagnose this, he would need to have a liver biopsy to which he agreed. Although a painful procedure, it is often the best way to definitively diagnose cirrhosis. Unfortunately, cirrhosis of the liver was confirmed. Bill was devastated. He was referred to a liver specialist, who told Bill that the only way to halt the progression of his liver disease and prevent liver failure, which could ultimately end his life, would be to stop drinking.

Bill returned to me with this news and we discussed a plan to turn his health around. I suggested to Bill that he would need to follow the 7-Day Liver Detox Diet for at least three months. I recommended he cut down alcohol over the next month to avoid withdrawal symptoms and then to have no alcohol for the next two months following this. I gave him a vitamin supplement containing B12 as well as thiamine, which is often deficient in those who drink heavily. I asked Bill to avoid red meat for this period of time to lower his iron levels. I impressed upon him the need to reduce his stress levels as they were the main trigger for his drinking, and suggested he see a counsellor to help with the alcohol addiction as well as his depression, to which he agreed.

When Bill returned for a review he reported that he really struggled to change his drinking habits. He had cut down alcohol to half of what he was having beforehand but was simply unable to quit. He had stuck to the new diet quite well with the occasional meal out at a restaurant. He had lost around 5kg and was feeling better for making some small changes. He had started walking with a small group three days a week for thirty minutes, which he said had really helped with his stress levels. I asked Bill to return in another two months' time following repeating his blood tests. I also asked that he continue to attempt to quit drinking and to consider joining a support group if he thought that may help to keep him accountable.

When Bill returned several months later he seemed a lot happier. He had found a new partner through his walking group who happened to be in the health industry and was very motivated to help Bill with his health. She had encouraged him to reduce his alcohol intake further and had continued to improve his diet. Bill was a much more confident man and no longer looked grey. He still had quite a lot of weight around his mid-section but had also lost some weight. His new blood results indicated that his liver damage was improving with his elevated liver markers nearly half of what they had been. His iron stores (ferritin) had reduced to 750 and his blood sugar and cholesterol levels were almost normal. I encouraged him to continue with his lifestyle change, obviously now supported by his new partner which made things easier. I mentioned that although the cirrhosis that he has is permanent he can prevent it from getting worse and can optimise the functioning of his remaining healthy liver tissue. He seemed happy with this plan and proud of his efforts, which I of course supported.

Liver Case #4 – Brave Enough to Change

Taylor is a 21-year-old woman who had recently moved away from family to start studying at university. She came to see me after being referred by one of her mother's friends who lived in the area. She was feeling tired all the time, had put on around 7kg of weight, and was finding it difficult to keep up with her university studies. Her symptoms had begun around 18 months ago after she broke up with her boyfriend of two years.

Since that time, Taylor said that she had started going out more often with friends and was partying every weekend. She was binge drinking to the point of either becoming unconscious or completely unaware of her behaviour most Friday and Saturday nights. She would then take around six paracetamol tablets throughout the following day to overcome a hangover headache so that she could work at her part-time job in a café. Throughout the week she rarely drank alcohol and was exercising three days a week. Her diet was quite high in refined sugars and processed foods as she rarely cooked for herself but ate convenience foods most of the time.

I examined Taylor and noticed that she had dark circles under her eyes and was very pale. She was slightly overweight and looked very unhealthy in general. When I felt her abdomen her liver and stomach regions were tender. Her blood pressure was normal.

I recommended to Taylor that she undergo some basic blood tests to see what might be the cause of her symptoms. Although she was quite needle-phobic she agreed. The results of her liver blood tests were the following:

- Total bilirubin 16 (normal)
- ALP 55 (normal)
- GGT 95 (elevated)
- ALT 365 (very elevated)
- AST 220 (very elevated)

Her iron stores were slightly elevated which is quite rare in young women who have regular menstrual periods. This indicated liver inflammation which leads to increased iron stores. Alarmingly her blood sugar levels were also markedly elevated as was her triglyceride levels (bad cholesterol). I asked her to have an oral glucose test to rule out diabetes. This was undertaken and she was confirmed insulin resistant (or pre-diabetes). Taylor did have a family history of diabetes but all her other family members had developed this at a later age.

Despite being shocked at the news, Taylor decided that this was the motivation she needed to change. I explained to her that she likely had acute alcoholic hepatitis from binge drinking, which was confirmed on liver ultrasound testing. She was going to need to be brave enough to say no to drinking on the weekends with friends, even if this meant finding a different social circle – the temptation to continue the same pattern of drinking would be too great. I suggested to Taylor to follow the 6-Step Liver Detox Plan and to keep up her exercise. She was also to avoid taking any paracetamol tablets, which were placing a further strain on her already damaged liver. I suggested perhaps seeing a counsellor or enlist a support person

to help her deal with having to change her lifestyle as well as to deal with any unsettled grief with her ex.

Taylor followed my suggestions and after four weeks returned for a review of her results. Overall she felt a lot better and had more energy. She looked less pasty in appearance and her abdomen was less bloated. She was finding the 6-Step Liver Detox Plan easy to follow and had not had a drink in four weeks, which to her surprise she said she didn't even miss. She said it was nice not to wake up with a hangover. Her repeat blood tests revealed that her liver markers had come down by about a third and that her blood glucose level and cholesterol had also reduced closer to an acceptable level. I mentioned to Taylor that she would need to continue this lifestyle change for at least another two months before drinking alcohol.

I saw Taylor three months later and she sheepishly admitted that she had been drinking again, although not as much as previously. She was in another relationship that was based around partying and drinking. She had gained another 2kg and was feeling pretty low. Although she had continued to stick to the 7-Day Liver Detox Diet she admitted that this had gone 'out the window' on the weekends. She had little energy for exercise and was finding it hard to sleep a full night as she was now needing to go to the bathroom several times a night to pass urine.

Taylor's repeat blood testing revealed that her liver markers had increased but were not as high as they had been. Unfortunately, however, Taylor had now developed type 2 diabetes. Although extremely rare in her age group I am seeing more young people develop this condition, which is devastating. I explained that her body had tipped over metabolically into an irreversible condition that she obviously had a genetic predisposition for. I encouraged her to delay its progression despite knowing she would have the diabetes for life, to prevent it from damaging her heart, kidneys and nerves. I encouraged her to continue to follow my initial suggestions but this time with increased reason.

Although devastated, Taylor accepted the news and decided to move back home to be closer to family support (and the healthy home cooking) and to get away from negative influences. The last time I heard from Taylor she was doing well and was continuing to make progress with her lifestyle changes.

Liver Case #5 – A Pain in the Guts

Sally is a 45-year-old single woman who had always put her career in sales first. She was usually very confident and prided herself in her appearance. She came to see me because in the last four months she had been experiencing a lot of pain in the right side of her abdomen, particularly after eating fatty foods. She had noticed that her abdomen was very bloated and that she often passed clay-coloured stools. Her urine had become darker in colour but did not smell particularly offensive. She had otherwise been well in the past with no obvious medical issues.

I asked Sally about her lifestyle and found that she was often required to take clients out for lunches at which she mostly chose to eat a Caesar salad. Lunch would often go for at least an hour and sometimes longer if a sales deal was involved and so it was not uncommon for Sally to share a bottle of wine or two with others at the table. This was often followed by after-work socialising and more drinks at least two nights of the week. Sally found the time in her week to walk most days and also did Pilates or yoga once or twice a week.

On examination, Sally was a little overweight but otherwise looked quite

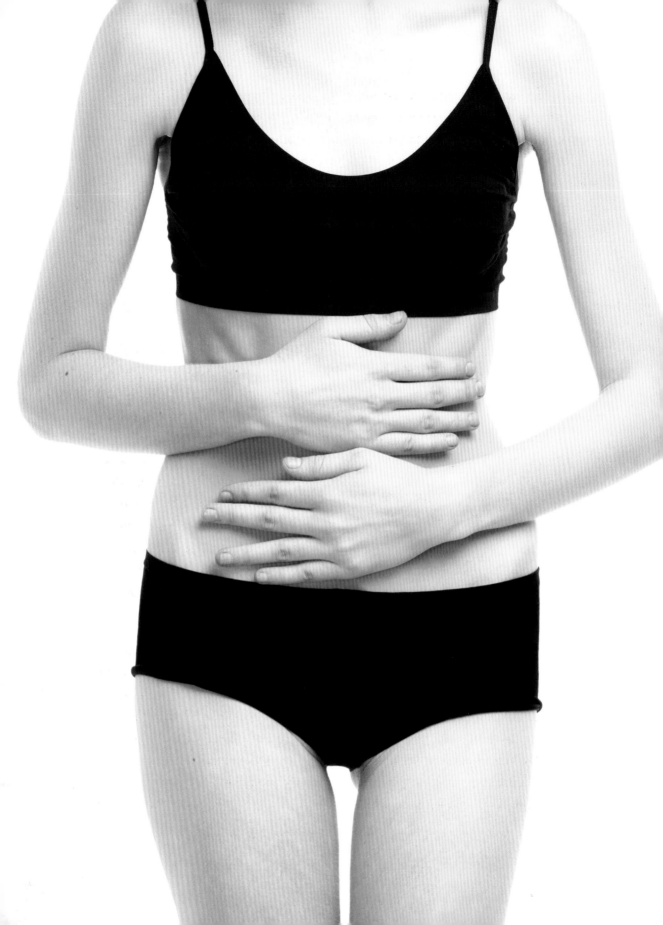

healthy. She had normal blood pressure. Her right upper abdomen was very tender particularly when I asked her to breathe in. She almost jumped off the bed and said that my placing pressure in this area had reproduced the pain that she was experiencing. I examined her face and skin and noticed that she appeared to be slightly jaundiced. She had not noticed this but admitted that since I'd mentioned it perhaps she could see that her complexion was slightly more yellow than usual.

I asked Sally to have a blood test done as well as a liver ultrasound, given the tenderness under her right ribs. The results revealed the following:

- Total bilirubin 45 (very elevated)

- ALP 125 (elevated)

- GGT 75 (slightly elevated)

- ALT 54 (slightly elevated)

- AST 45 (slightly elevated)

Her other blood test results were in the normal range including her pancreatic enzyme markers (the pancreas can become inflamed as a result of gallbladder disease). Her liver ultrasound revealed that she had gallstones and was at risk of an acute gallbladder infection due to the size and position of the gallstones. This condition can be extremely painful and is often the reason why surgeons will recommend removal of the gallbladder in order to prevent this from happening.

I explained the results to Sally and told her that the gallstones were causing the pain she was feeling as well as inflaming her liver. I mentioned that these had been caused by her lifestyle – principally a diet rich in saturated and processed fats and sugars as well as too much alcohol. I recommended that she follow my 7-Day Liver Detox Diet for at least two weeks and avoid all alcohol. I gave her healthier options for dining out and suggested she sip on mineral water instead of wine at lunch. Although a little reluctant, Sally agreed. She did not want the pain to return. I did warn Sally that if she did get another gallbladder attack that she may need surgery. This was the final motivation she needed to stick to my suggestions.

When Sally returned for a review several weeks later she reported that she was no longer experiencing pain and that she felt a lot better for it. She even thought she may have lost a kilogram or two and so was happy to continue her new lifestyle if it meant that these positive changes were going to continue. We repeated her blood testing a month later and it showed that her levels had returned to normal. Although the gallstones were still present they were not getting any bigger. She decided not to have preventative removal of her gallbladder but, rather, waited to see if she got any further gallbladder 'attacks'. The last time I saw Sally, which was twelve months after she initially came to see me, she had not had any gallbladder pains and was sticking to my suggestions and allowing herself to have the occasional glass of wine.

Liver Case #6 – A Bygone Life Leaves its Mark

Adam is a 44-year-old man who recently got married and was sent in to see me by his wife. He had been feeling more tired than usual over the last few months and was finding it hard to cope with the long hours he did at work. As a plasterer he was often up by 4:30 am to get to construction sites early and was home by 4pm. Until recently he had been running and swimming and was hoping to compete in a fundraising team triathlon event later in the year. He was finding lately, however, that he was unable to do any training due to fatigue.

Adam was otherwise healthy, although he admitted that he had not had a medical check-up by a doctor for 'as long as he could remember'. He had no family history of any health conditions as far as he knew and he himself did not have any significant medical history. He stuck to a healthy diet and only drunk in moderation on the weekends by having one or two beers at barbeques with friends. He hadn't noticed any other symptoms other than fatigue. He denied any symptoms of depression or insomnia, which can sometimes mask other health conditions.

On examination Adam's blood pressure was normal and he was a healthy weight for his build. He was slightly pale and looked fatigued with dark circles under his eyes. His abdomen was slightly tender under his right ribs but was otherwise normal. I asked Adam to have some initial blood testing to see what might be the issue.

He returned for the results which were as follows:

- Total bilirubin 19 (normal)

- ALP 45 (normal)

- GGT 60 (normal)

- ALT 1250 (very elevated)

- AST 1800 (very elevated)

His ferritin level (iron stores) were also elevated at 450 indicating liver inflammation. His white cell count, particularly his lymphocyte count (a marker of viral infection) was slightly elevated as was his inflammatory markers known as CRP and ESR. As these results pointed to acute liver infection with a virus, I asked Adam whether he had been unwell with flu-like symptoms. He said he hadn't. I asked whether he had travelled overseas recently and picked up food poisoning, which he also said that he hadn't. I queried his risk of having any other viruses such as hepatitis. I also asked him whether he had any tattoos. Although he did have several tattoos on his torso he claimed they had been done in a fairly sterile environment. He did admit, though, that when he was in his twenties and early thirties he had injected drugs intravenously. He had been heavily addicted for several years until deciding to get help. He was able to kick the habit and didn't think much of it after this.

I then ran a few tests for hepatitis C, hepatitis B and HIV infections. Luckily he was negative for the latter two infections but did come back positive for hepatitis C infection. His viral load, which is a test for how much virus is currently active in his system, was moderately elevated explaining why his liver was so inflamed

and why he was feeling so tired. Hepatitis C is transmitted by blood and is quite common in intravenous drug users, particularly those who share or reuse needles. It causes liver inflammation and can lead to liver cancer.

Of course Adam was distraught at the news, not knowing what his long-term prognosis would be and he was also worried for his wife's health. He had no idea that he carried this illness and had thought that he had been checked for it previously at a sexual health clinic. I explained that hepatitis C, as with hepatitis B and HIV, can remain latent in the system and can be difficult to detect until viral levels are high enough to be identified in the blood. I explained that it was passed via blood products and not typically sexually transmitted, so his wife should be safe although caution was needed not to share blood – such as avoiding using each others' toothbrushes or razors.

I mentioned to Adam that he would need to see an infectious diseases specialist to determine a hepatitis C treatment for him, which was his best chance at inducing remission from the illness and could in some cases result in a cure. I suggested to Adam that he follow the 7-Day Liver Detox Diet but increase the protein content of his main meals as his liver wold likely require the extra protein to heal. I also suggested to him that alongside his anti-viral medication he should also take a higher dose of vitamin C, zinc and selenium as well as St Mary's Thistle.

Adam started anti-viral treatment and although he felt very run down whilst on the treatment he recovered well from it afterwards. Fortunately for Adam he had the type of Hepatitis C virus (there are at least six subtypes) that responds well to treatment. After twelve months of treatment he seemed to have been cured of the illness. He was very grateful that the virus had been found early enough to do something about it. This case explains the importance of having regular medical check-ups even if you feel relatively well.

Liver Case #7 – A Case of Missing Periods

Madison is a 27-year-old woman who first came to see me wanting to start a family. She had been married for three months and had never been pregnant previously. She mentioned that she had always had good health up until around six months ago when the stress of the wedding planning and work responsibilities were

'all getting a bit too much'. She felt tired in the afternoons and often needed a nap on the weekends, had gained around 3kg since the wedding, and was craving a lot more sugar than she used to. Madison had stopped taking the oral contraceptive pill around eight months before, thinking that it may take awhile to restore her menstrual cycles but as yet hadn't had a menstrual period. Prior to starting the oral contraceptive pill at age 17, Madison had always had regular periods. Since stopping the pill she noticed that she was getting a bit of acne along her jawline and chin, which she had never had in the past. Her PAP test the previous year had been normal and she had never had any gynaecology issues in the past.

I examined Madison and found that she was slightly overweight for her frame but generally appeared healthy. She had a normal blood pressure and no fluid retention. Her abdomen was soft with no tenderness. I then asked Madison to have some initial blood tests including hormone and liver function tests. I also asked her to have a pelvic ultrasound to make sure that her uterus and ovaries were anatomically normal.

Madison returned two weeks later for the results. Her hormone blood test revealed that she wasn't ovulating but that there was no sign of premature menopause. Her iron levels were normal as was her vitamin B12 and folate level, which ruled them out as the cause of her fatigue. Her thyroid function testing was also normal. Her liver function testing, however, revealed the following:

- Total bilirubin 19 (normal)

- ALP 45 (normal)

- GGT 60 (normal)

- ALT 57 (slightly elevated)

- AST 62 (slightly elevated)

As Madison was a non-drinker and had no other obvious cause for the elevation in her liver function testing I suspected polycystic ovary syndrome. This would explain the lack of menstrual periods and was subsequently confirmed on the ultrasound test, which showed that Madison had several cysts on her ovaries.

Polycystic ovary syndrome is a relatively common condition affecting one in ten women. Many women do not realise they have this condition but it is a common cause of irregular menstrual periods, acne, weight gain and infertility. Most women discover that they have this condition when they come off the oral contraceptive pill because, just like Madison, that's when symptoms start to show.

The other common problem that I see with polycystic ovary syndrome is that insulin resistance can start to develop. This is a condition whereby the body becomes less able to regulate its blood sugar levels. Weight gain, sugar cravings and liver issues often then result. This of course is not in all cases, but I do see it in the majority. This is especially the case if stress and/or poor lifestyle choices are thrown in the mix as as was the case with Madison.

I explained the results to Madison and how her polycystic ovaries were causing her symptoms. I explained that this was likely causing issues with her blood sugar levels, making her feel tired and making her gain weight. I also explained that with this condition hormone imbalance can occur, which results in irregular periods and acne. Madison naturally felt overwhelmed at what this may mean for her fertility and ability to have children. I explained that in some cases extra support with fertility medications may be required but by and large many of her symptoms should resolve with some lifestyle changes.

I suggested to Madison that she follow the 7-Day Liver Detox Diet for one month and that she ideally not have any alcohol in this time. She was to work on reducing her sugar intake as prescribed in the 6-Step Liver Detox Plan as large amounts of sugar intake would worsen her symptoms. I recommended that she start exercising regularly and building up her lean muscle tissue by doing some resistance training – body weight exercise to begin and then building to light weight training. Muscle tissue helps to burn sugar and would help to stabilise her blood sugar levels.

I also suggested that Madison take some supportive supplements, primarily St Mary's Thistle, zinc and a B vitamin complex containing vitamins B1, B3, B6, P5P (activated B6), B12 and activated folate to help support her energy levels. I also recommended she start a pregnancy supplement 'just in case' she fell pregnant. Additionally, she was prescribed a supplement to help support healthy hormone balance – one containing indole-3-carbinol.

Madison returned several weeks later to report that she was doing well. She still hadn't had a menstrual period but was feeling better. She was less tired and bloated and her acne had also started to clear. She was yet to lose weight but had not yet begun exercising, which she planned to start in the coming week with a personal trainer.

Several months later when Madison returned she excitedly reported that she was seven weeks pregnant. She had had one normal menstrual period and then fell pregnant that next cycle. She was coping well with the pregnancy and was continuing to eat a healthy diet, following the principles of the 7-Day Liver Detox Diet but with increased protein, calcium and iron to meet pregnancy requirements. I asked her to stop her supplements except her pregnancy supplement as the others were no longer needed. Madison eventually gave birth to a healthy baby boy.

This case highlights how sometimes our bodies don't reflect certain symptoms of an underlying condition we may have – particular circumstances, such as high stress levels, reveal what is happening. This drives home how important it is to have regular medical check-ups to make sure that we aren't overlooking our health, thinking that our symptoms are normal or will resolve.

►►►

LOVE YOUR LIVER FOR LIFE

▼▼▼▼▼▼▼▼▼▼▼▼▼▼▼▼▼▼▼▼▼▼▼▼▼▼▼▼▼
·····································

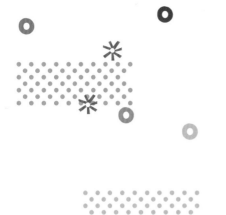

As we arrive at the end of this book you have hopefully come to fully understand what your liver does and how important it is for good health. Congratulations on completing this journey and undertaking the challenge to truly detox your liver by following Your Liver Detox Plan. You should be proud of yourself. And even though you may have thought that you had no choice but to do something about your health, many people find it so difficult to take the first step that they do nothing at all. So well done on taking action!

By now you should be able to recognise symptoms of poor liver health and understand how the liver may be damaged by everyday choices that we make. Hopefully you now feel empowered to be able to do something, whether it be correcting long-term neglect or changing your habits like those weekend-long indulgences.

For ease of reference a list of these important areas has been provided in the final section of this book. In this section you will find a recap of the list of 'Liver Haters' – substances that damage the liver and should be avoided and 'Liver Lovers' – substances that help to heal and support the liver. There is also a 'Liver-Friendly Shopping List' – a list of foods to purchase as part of Your Liver Detox or maintenance plan, and a summary of Your Liver Detox Plan as well as a recap of Your Post-Party Detox. Feel free to photocopy these and place them on the refrigerator or take a photo of them on your phone for quick reference when out shopping or dining.

Finally, my hope and wish is that you continue to love your liver, not just in the short-term when your symptoms are acute, but for life. As you experience the benefits of a healthy liver remember to bring others on the journey with you and to share what you have learnt. So many of us can benefit from what you now know. A healthier, more energised life will be their reward for following this advice.

All my very best for your health for years to come!

EASY
REFERENCE
GUIDE

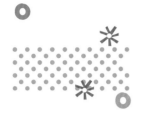

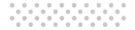

- Alcohol

- Heavy metals e.g. mercury, aluminium, cadmium, lead and copper

- Many artificial food additives

- Certain medications such as paracetamol, and certain antibiotics and anti-fungal medications.

LIVER HATERS LIST

The following is a list of substances that can damage the liver:

Toxins:

- *Exotoxins* – are toxins found in our outside environment and include:

  - Industrial pollution

  - Agricultural pesticides (may be residual on unwashed produce)

  - Some cleaning products

  - Plastics e.g. bisphenol-A (BPA) found in some food storage containers, baby bottles and plastic toys and plastic cutlery

  - Cigarette smoke

  - Recreational drugs

Overload Agents:

- Fructose

- Refined carbohydrates

- Processed, unhealthy fats

- Iron rich foods when the liver is already inflamed

Micro-organisms:

- Blood-borne Hepatitis viruses – Hepatitis C and B (transmitted by blood and other body fluids)

- Food-borne Hepatitis viruses – Hepatitis A, E (transmitted via contaminated food)

- Food-borne bacteria – E.coli, salmonella, campylobacter. These are found in contaminated food such as undercooked chicken.

- HIV

- Malaria

- Tuberculosis

- Epstein-Barr Virus (EBV) and Cytomegalovirus (CMV). EBV causes glandular fever.

Conditions of the Liver

The following conditions can be a result of significant damage to the liver by the above substances:

- Fatty liver disease

- Metabolic syndrome

- Hepatitis

- Cirrhosis

- Acute liver inflammation

- Gallbladder and/or bile duct disease

LIVER LOVERS LIST

The following is a list of liver-loving substances that can be included in your everyday life to support and help heal the liver:

Liver Loving Foods

- Vegetables from the 'brassica' family – broccoli, kale, cauliflower, Brussels sprouts and cabbage. Eating a serve of these types of vegetables regularly will help give your liver a boost.

- Fruits containing ellagic acid such as raspberries and red grapes

- Spices including garlic, onion, rosemary, fennel and turmeric

- Dandelion – often found in tea form. Include up to several cups of dandelion tea per day.

- Proteins – the liver needs quality proteins to function optimally. Good protein sources include lean meats, legumes, beans and wholegrains such as quinoa, buckwheat and millet.

- Green tea – has been shown to support liver detoxification. Remember, though, that green tea contains caffeine so avoid having more than two to three cups per day.

Liver Loving Lifestyles

- Remember moderation with eating – 80:20 rule.

- Watch alcohol – One standard drink five days a week for women and two standard drinks five days a week for men. Keep alcohol-free days consecutive.

- Reduce caffeine – keep it to a maximum of 3-4 cups of tea or coffee per day, which also includes caffeinated herbal teas such as white tea, oolong and green tea.

- Include exercise as part of your weekly routine – aim for thirty minutes most days per week.

Liver Loving Supplements

For a list of specific supplements and dosages to suit your liver and for liver health refer to Step Four – 'Choose Liver Supplements Wisely' of the 6-Step Liver Detox Plan listed below.

Herbs	Schizandra, St John's wort, rosemary, milk thistle, turmeric, dandelion root
Antioxidants	Coenzyme Q10, bioflavonoids, alpha lipoic acid.
Vitamins	The antioxidant vitamins A, C and E as well as thiamin (B1), niacin (B3), pyridoxine (B6), B12 and folic acid.
Minerals	Zinc, selenium, manganese, magnesium
Amino acids	Cysteine, glutathione, L-glycine, L-glutamine, taurine, and methylation cofactors. Because glutathione is poorly absorbed from the digestive tract it is often given as N-acetyl cysteine (NAC).

LIVER SYMPTOM TRACKER

Use the below tracker to gauge your symptoms as you go through the 7-Day Liver Detox Diet. Tick the symptom as it applies. Notice as you go further along in the detox process how the number of negative symptoms reduces and number of positive symptoms increase.

Symptom	Day 1	Day 2	Day 3	Day 4	Day 5	Day 6	Day 7
Negative Symptoms							
Headaches							
Bloating							
Indigestion							
Nausea							
Dizziness							
Bad Breath							
Irritability							
Fatigue							
Constipation							
Diarrhoea							
Fluid Retention							
Poor Sleep							
Blotchy Skin							

Symptom	Day 1	Day 2	Day 3	Day 4	Day 5	Day 6	Day 7
Positive Symptoms							
Clear Eyes							
Better Concentration							
Better Memory							
Clear Skin							
No Tongue Coating							
Improved Sleep							
Less Bloating							
Better Mood							
Less Headaches							
More Energy							

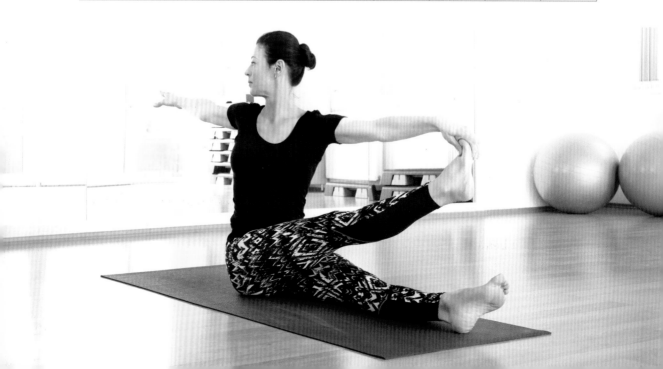

LIVER-FRIENDLY SHOPPING LIST

The following foods are to be included as part of your 7-Day Liver Detox Diet. Choose any of the foods from the below list when you are grocery shopping. Stock a variety of foods in your pantry or refrigerator so that they are at hand when you are hungry or need to prepare a meal. Also check the 'Avoid' category to make sure you are not stocking anything that is bad for your liver.

Protein Options

- ✓ Chicken
- ✓ Eggs
- ✓ Fresh fish (except shellfish or shark, orange roughy, swordfish and ling)
- ✓ Calamari
- ✓ Tempeh or tofu
- ✓ Turkey

Beans & Legume Options

- ✓ Broad beans
- ✓ Borlotti beans
- ✓ Butter beans
- ✓ Kidney beans
- ✓ Chickpeas
- ✓ Lima beans
- ✓ Pinto beans
- ✓ Black beans
- ✓ Navy beans
- ✓ Split peas
- ✓ Lentils
- ✓ Adzuki beans
- ✓ Alfalfa sprouts

Grains & Starch Options

- ✓ Brown or wild rice
- ✓ Buckwheat
- ✓ Millet
- ✓ Quinoa
- ✓ Amaranth
- ✓ Traditional or steel cut oats (not instant)
- ✓ Corn
- ✓ Gluten-free flours made from the above

- ✓ Gluten-free rice or corn cakes or crackers (unflavoured)

- ✓ Almond or hazelnut meals

- ✓ Coconut flour

Vegetable Options

- ✓ All vegetables (except potato)

- ✓ All salad greens

- ✓ Fermented vegetables including sauerkraut or kimchi (organic preferably)

Fruit Options

- ✓ All fresh fruits

- ✓ Frozen berries

Dairy & Dairy Alternative Options

- ✓ Unsweetened brown rice milk or nut milks

- ✓ Goat's or sheep's milk

- ✓ Unhomogenised cow's milk (A2 preferably)

- ✓ Plain unsweetened yoghurt

Nuts & Seed Options

- ✓ Almonds (around 20 almonds per day)

- ✓ Brazil nuts (limit to 5 per day)

- ✓ Chia seeds

- ✓ Coconut

- ✓ Hazelnuts

- ✓ Linseeds/flaxseeds

- ✓ Macadamia nuts

- ✓ Pecans

- ✓ Pepitas

- ✓ Pine nuts

- ✓ Sesame seeds

- ✓ Sunflower seeds

- ✓ Walnuts

Oil Options (for cooking)

- ✓ Macadamia oil

- ✓ Flaxseed (linseed) oil

- ✓ Rice bran oil

- ✓ Sesame oil

- ✓ Grape seed oil

- ✓ Walnut oil

- ✓ Coconut oil

Oil Options (for dressings)
- ✓ Olive oil
- ✓ Avocado oil

Herbs, Spices, & Condiment Options
- ✓ Any natural herbs and spices
- ✓ Garlic
- ✓ Himalayan or Celtic sea salt
- ✓ Black or cayenne pepper
- ✓ Lemon juice
- ✓ Apple cider vinegar
- ✓ Red or white wine vinegar
- ✓ Organic tamari
- ✓ Balsamic vinegar
- ✓ Mustard
- ✓ Tahini
- ✓ Stevia and/or xylitol
- ✓ Honey
- ✓ Rice bran or rice malt syrup

Drinks
- ✓ Herbal tea (non-caffeinated) – try Tulsi tea, chamomile, dandelion or peppermint
- ✓ Green tea or oolong tea
- ✓ Sparling mineral water

Other Items
- ✓ Psyllium husks (for added fibre)
- ✓ Pea or brown rice protein

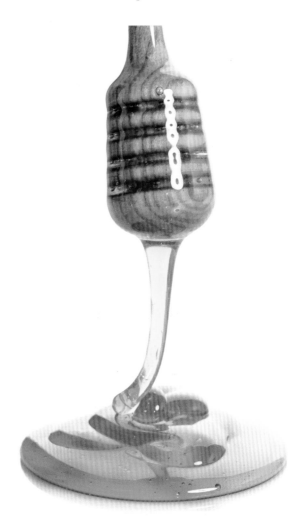

YOUR 6-STEP LIVER DETOX SUMMARY

The below diagram summarises the steps involved in Your Liver Detox Plan as outlined fully in the corresponding chapter of this book.

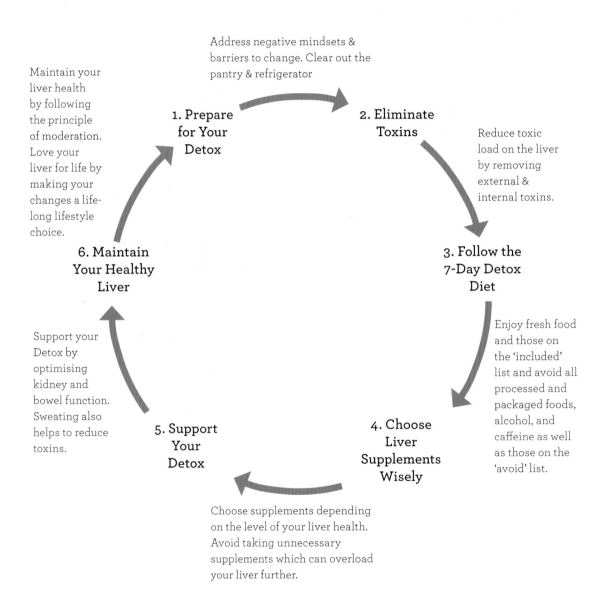

Address negative mindsets & barriers to change. Clear out the pantry & refrigerator

1. Prepare for Your Detox

2. Eliminate Toxins

Reduce toxic load on the liver by removing external & internal toxins.

Maintain your liver health by following the principle of moderation. Love your liver for life by making your changes a life-long lifestyle choice.

6. Maintain Your Healthy Liver

3. Follow the 7-Day Detox Diet

Enjoy fresh food and those on the 'included' list and avoid all processed and packaged foods, alcohol, and caffeine as well as those on the 'avoid' list.

Support your Detox by optimising kidney and bowel function. Sweating also helps to reduce toxins.

5. Support Your Detox

4. Choose Liver Supplements Wisely

Choose supplements depending on the level of your liver health. Avoid taking unnecessary supplements which can overload your liver further.

YOUR POST-PARTY DETOX SUMMARY

Follow these simple tips for at least forty-eight hours after a party to help your body and liver recover and get back on track:

Step One – Reduce Toxic Fats

Avoid processed foods and meats, which contain high amounts of harmful fats. These fats can lead to liver disease as well as heart disease.

Step Two – Hydrate Well

Keep hydrated by drinking at least 2-3L of water per day. This aids liver detoxification and toxin elimination. Add lemon to your water if you prefer the taste and take a water bottle with you wherever you go.

Step Three – Avoid Alcohol

Avoid drinking any more alcohol in order to give your liver a break.

Step Four – Cut Back on Sugar

Avoid high amounts of fruit sugar and hidden sugars by keeping processed foods to a minimum. Excessive sugar intake can overwhelm the liver and contribute to fatty liver disease. Avoid dried fruit and fruit juices, which increase fruit sugar intake.

Step Five – Avoid Paracetamol

Avoid overloading your liver further and refrain from taking paracetamol, even if you have a hangover headache.

Step Six – Stay Regular

Avoid constipation by increasing fibre in your diet. This aids liver function through effective elimination.

HANGOVER DETOX GUIDE

Follow these simple steps to help your liver recover from a hangover quicker:

Step One - Start your morning with a large glass of water

Step Two - Eat a high-protein breakfast

Step Three - Eat a lighter lunch

Step Four - Trade coffee for herbal tea

Step Five - Make your evening meal the smallest of the day

Step Six - Avoid dessert

References

1 National Center for Health Statistics. National Vital Statistics Report. *Chronic liver disease/cirrhosis.* Accessed Jan 5, 2016, at: www.cdc.gov/nchs/fastats/liverdis.htm.

2 Dart RC, Erdman AR, Olson KR, Christianson G, Manoguerra AS, Chyka PA, et al. 2006. *Acetaminophen poisoning: an evidence-based consensus guideline for out-of-hospital management.* Clin Toxicol (Phila). 44(1):1-18.

3 Thomas C, Stevenson M, Riley TV. 2003. *Antibiotics and hospital-acquired Clostridium difficile-associated diarrhoea: a systematic review.* J. Antimicrob. Chemother. 51:1339-1350.

4 Bedogni G, Miglioli L, Masutti F, Tiribelli C, Marchesini G, Bellentani S. 2005. *Prevalence of and risk factors for nonalcoholic fatty liver disease: the Dionysos nutrition and liver study.* Hepatology. 42:44-52.

5 Paschos P & Paletas K. 2009. *Non alcoholic fatty liver disease and metabolic syndrome.* Hippokratia. 13(1): 9-19.

6 Bayram C, Valenti L, Miller G. 2013. *The right upper quadrant.* Australian Family Physician. 42 (7): 443-443.

7 Sweeney B, Vora M, Ulbricht C, Basch E. *Evidence-based systematic review of dandelion (Taraxacum officinale) by Natural Standard Research Collaboration.* J Herb Pharmacother. 2005;5(1):79-93.

8 Imai K, Nakachi K. *Cross sectional study of effects of drinking green tea on cardiovascular and liver diseases.* 1995. Br Med J Clin Res. 310:693-6.

9 Lawrence, G. 2013. *Dietary Fats and Health: Dietary Recommendations in the Context of Scientific Evidence.* Adv Nutr 4: 294-302.

10 Débora E et. Al. 2013. *Lipotoxicity: Effects of Dietary Saturated and Transfatty Acids.* Mediators of Inflammation, vol. 2013.

11 Simopoulos. 2008. *The Importance of the Omega-6/Omega-3 Fatty Acid Ratio in Cardiovascular Disease and Other Chronic Diseases.* Exp Biol Med (Maywood). 233 (6): 674-688.

12 Australian Government Department of Health. 2013. *Reduce your risk: new national guidelines for alcohol consumption* accessed Jan 10, 2016, at: http://www.alcohol.gov.au/internet/alcohol/publishing.nsf/Content/guide-adult.

13 Cavin, C. et al. 2008. *Induction of Nrf2-mediated cellular defenses and alteration of phase I activities as mechanisms of chemoprotective effects of coffee in the liver.* Food and Chemical Toxicology. 46(4): 1239-1248.

14 Acheson, K. 1980. *Caffeine and coffee: their influence on metabolic rate and substrate utilization in normal weight and obese individuals.* Am J Clin Nutr. 33 (5): 989-997.

15 Powell, N. et al. 2013. *Social stress up-regulates inflammatory gene expression in the leukocyte transcriptome via beta-adrenergic induction of myelopoiesis.* Proc Natl Acad Sci U S A. 110(41): 16574-16579.

16 Phelps, K and Hassad, C. *General Practice The Integrative Approach.* 2011. Elsevier Australia.

17 Pietrzykowska, N. 2016. *Benefits of 5-10 Percent Weight-loss.* Obesity Action Coalition. Accessed Jan 15, 2016, at: http://www.obesityaction.org/educational-resources/resource-articles-2/general-articles/benefits-of-5-10-percent-weight-loss.

18 Brennan, D. 2015. *The Facts About Bisphenol A.* WebMD. Accessed Jan 20, 2016, at: http://www.webmd.com/children/environmental-exposure-head2toe/bpa?page=3.

19 Bernardo, J. 2015. Aluminum Toxicity. Medscape. Accessed Jan 16, 2016, at: http://emedicine.medscape.com/article/165315-overview.

20 Sathyapalan, T. et al. 2011. *The Effect of Soy Phytoestrogen Supplementation on Thyroid Status and Cardiovascular Risk Markers in Patients with Subclinical Hypothyroidism: A Randomized, Double-Blind, Crossover Study.* J Clin Endo & Met. 96(5): 1442-1449.

21 Sears M, Kerr K. & Bray R. 2012. *Arsenic, Cadmium, Lead, and Mercury in Sweat: A Systematic Review.* J Environ & Public Health, vol. 2012.

22 Singh, S. et. Al. 2015. *Alcohol, glycine, and gastritis.* Innt J Nut Pharm Neuro Disease. 5(1): 1-5.

23 Crews, F et al. 2006. *Cytokines and alcohol.* Alcohol Clin Exp Res. 30(4):720-30.

24 Penning, R. et al. 2010. *The Pathology of Hangover.* Current Drug Abuse Reviews. 3 (2): 68-75.

A Rockpool book
PO Box 252
Summer Hill, NSW 2130, Australia
www.rockpoolpublishing.com.au
http://www.facebook.com/RockpoolPublishing

First published in 2016
Copyright © Dr Cris Beer 2016

ISBN 978-1-925017-57-1

A CIP catalogue record for this book is available from the National Library of Australia

Cover and internal design by Jessica Le
Editor: Katie Evans
Author Photographs by Bek Grace Photography
Photography on pages 84, 89, 91, 95, 97, 100, 103, 105, 107, 109 by Jason Malouin
Food styling by Brittany Lindores, The Foodie Chain, www.thefoodiechain.com.au
All other images from Shutterstock
Illustrations on pages 19, 33 by www.integraldms.com
Printed and bound in China
10 9 8 7 6 5 4 3 2 1